Adopting A Healthy Lifestyle

For An Active Body and Mind

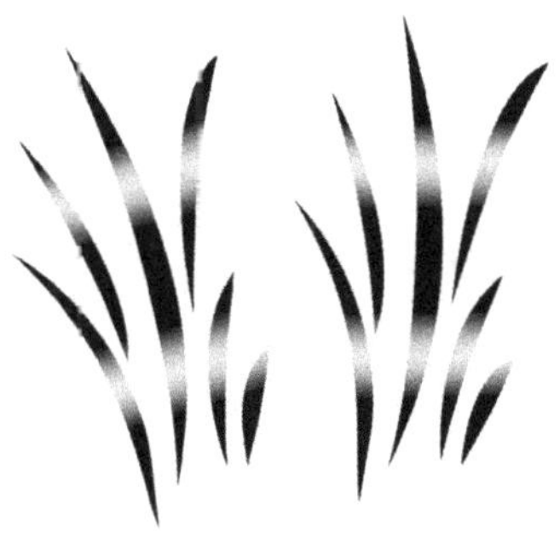

Adopting
A Healthy Lifestyle

For An Active Body and Mind

C.T. Pam

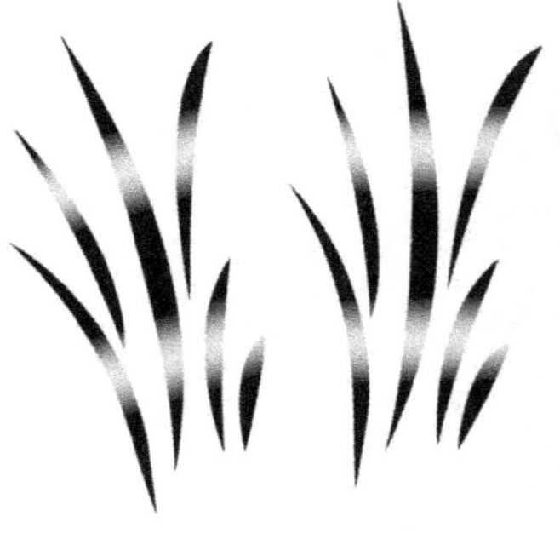

Published and printed in the United States by Innovative Publishers, Inc., Boston, Massachusetts.

Library of Congress Control Number: 2012954707

ISBN 13: 9781884711343
ISBN 10: 1-884711-34-0 Adopting a healthy lifestyle Paperback

Also available in the following formats

ISBN 13: 9781884711336 Kindle
ISBN 10: 1-884711-33-2

ISBN 13: 9781884711350 Hardback
ISBN 10: 1-884711-35-9

ISBN 13: 9781884711367 Audiobook
ISBN 10: 1-884711-36-7

ISBN 13: 9781884711374 iBook
ISBN 10: 1-884711-37-5

ISBN 13: 9781884711442 Nook
ISBN 10: 1-884711-44-8

Printed in the United States of America
10 9 8 7 6 5 4 3 2 1 13 14 15 16

First edition, January 2013

For general information on our other products and services or for technical support, please contact our technical support within the United States at pub@innovative-publishers.com or fax # 617-861-8533.

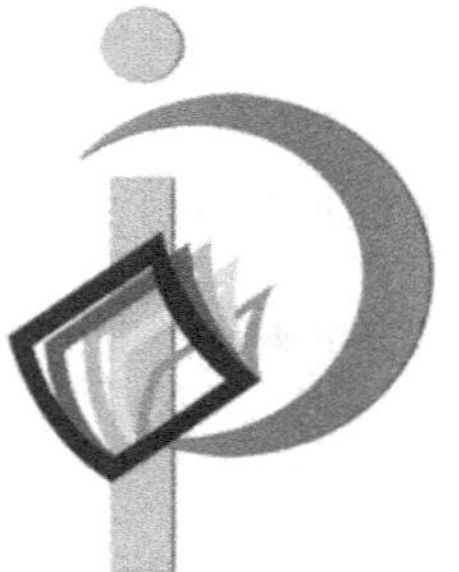

Innovative Publishers

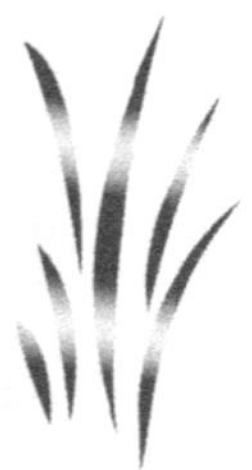

Contents

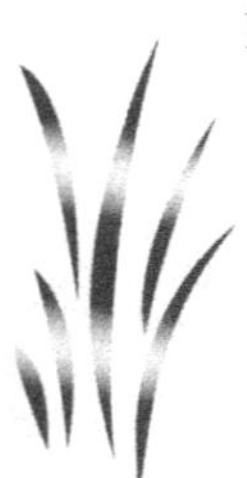

Introduction to Weight Management

With the rapid rate at which obesity has spread over the last couple of decades, the importance of weight management programs has also grown as a consequence. Weight management program refers to all those activities that help an individual to either gain weight, lose weight or even to maintain it at the current level. In any of these goals, a weight management program targets increasing or maintaining the amount of lean muscle mass while decreasing the body fat percentage. Any other way of losing or gaining weight will be unhealthy in one aspect or another and may compromise health in the short term, but definitely in the long run.

Body Composition

Our body comprises of different components, namely fat, lean muscle, water, bones, organs etc. Each of them contributes to the total body weight. For each and every individual each of these constituent elements is present in different proportions. The ratio in which this distribution is present in any individual is called body composition. In the context of weight management, the division is done into two categories – fat mass and fat free mass. A healthy body composition is one in which the fat mass is low and fat free mass is higher. Through different weight management programs it is attempted to alter body composition in a manner that it boosts good health.

There are many techniques and methods to determine body composition. With technological advancements newer and more accurate equipments are available for performing body composition analysis. Traditional techniques such as skin fold measurements are easy to implement but have limited accuracy. Newer technologies such as ultrasound and bioelectric impedance analysis help in doing body composition analysis using simple and portable machines that give extremely accurate results as well. These different methods determine not only the amount of fat and lean muscle tissue but also provide a segmental analysis so that appropriate intervention strategies can be planned as part of the weight management program.

Doing body composition analysis on a regular basis should be included as part of any weight management strategy since it will help in monitoring the alterations taking place in the body as a result of the program. Since the body is undergoing change on a regular basis it is imperative that the program should also change accordingly. A program that was designed for the individual who weighed say 240 pounds will need to be changed when the person loses weight and weighs 200 pounds now. Body composition analysis also provides information on whether the weight loss is happening in a healthy manner or not. In case the weight loss happens at the expense of lean muscle or water then changes need to be done in the program so that these components can be restored to normal levels and fat loss targeted by introducing appropriate changes. A number of new age weight loss methods as well as gadgets are able to provide good results in terms of weight loss but they do it at the expense of good health. Doing a simple body composition analysis will reveal the true nature of these unhealthy methods and systems. Most new technologies also provide information on metabolic rate which is directly correlated the amount of lean mass in the body. Greater the lean mass higher will be the energy that is required by the body to maintain it. The measurement of metabolic rate helps in designing the exercise program as well as the calorie intake required as part of the diet & nutrition plan. Since the needs and requirement of each and every individual are different, the weight management strategy has to be necessarily different as well. Body composition analysis is the first step in designing a weight management program and should thereafter be done on a regular basis.

Problems with Adverse Body Composition

A body composition analysis that reveals high fat percentage in comparison to lean muscle mass percentage points to obesity. Obesity is a modern day lifestyle disease that is essentially a silent killer. It indirectly leads to other physical as well as mental disorders, ailments and diseases that later on deplete the quality of life of the individual and in certain cases may even lead to death. The most common ailments that accompany obesity include type-2 diabetes, hypertension, cardiovascular & coronary artery disease, metabolic syndrome polycystic ovary syndrome and Dyslipidemia. Obesity also leads to gastrointestinal issues such as Cholelithiasis, GERD or Gastroesophageal Reflex Disease, Fatty Liver Disease, Colon Cancer and Hernia; genitourinary problems include erectile dysfunction, renal failure, incontinence and hypogonadism; Respiratory problems include sleep apnea, Hypoventilation syndrome and dyspnea. Apart from these physical ailments obesity also leads to psychological problems that arise from a diminished self confidence and if left unchecked may even lead to chronic depression.

Causes of Obesity

Obesity is caused by an energy intake in the form of diet that is not balanced by equivalent amount of physical activity. The basic law of conservation of energy cannot be violated at any cost and hence, energy excess will lead to weight gain while energy deficit will lead to weight loss. Energy input into the body is through the food that we eat. Energy output is the sum of a number of parameters that include – energy expended through physical exercise, energy spent in activities performed in daily life, basal metabolic rate or the energy required by the body to perform essential body functions such as respiration and digestion; in addition there are a few other parameters such as *thermic effect of food* and *adaptive thermogenesis* that add onto energy output but only in relatively small amounts. It is when the energy input becomes greater than energy output that the body starts storing this excess energy in the form of body fat. Some amount of fat is essential for efficient body functioning but when the fat percentage goes above certain levels it leads to obesity and consequently a host of other disorders and diseases.

This energy imbalance is the objective reason behind obesity but it is important to understand the underlying reasons why this imbalance is created. Imbalanced diet and sedentary lifestyle are the primary causes which get accentuated as a result of numerous personal, social, cultural and familial issues. Genetics and medical conditions also contribute towards increasing the fat mass in an individual. While most parameters seem to be alterable, some of these parameters may not seem to be in control of the individual and a situation of helplessness may be experienced. However, there are ways and means to counter any of these issues that gradually lead to weight loss in a healthy manner.

Genetic Factors and Body Type

As mentioned above certain parameters that influence body composition cannot be modified. Genetic predisposition is one such parameter. Genetics define the body type of an individual which then affects the way in which the body reacts to a certain lifestyle and also to any alteration that is forced on this lifestyle. There are different classification techniques for differentiating between different body types.

1. The ancient Indian science of *Ayurveda* uses a classification method based on energy patterns or types. It is believed as per *Ayurveda* that the universe comprises of five basic elements – space, air, water, fire and earth. A combination of these basic elements is responsible for defining the human physiology. The basis of classification therefore is on the basis of energy patterns or *doshas* which comprise of one or more of these elements. The three *doshas – vata, pitta* and *kapha* define the person's physiology and all *Ayurvedic* treatments start from the identification of the *dosha* and identifying the imbalance in the *dosha* pattern. Once this is done remedial solution can be prescribed the aim of which is to restore the balance in the elements.
2. The second classification technique is based on the metabolic type. Under this classification technique the basis of differentiation between body types is the dominating gland in the endocrine system. It is believed that the biochemical reactions happening in the body of the individual are influenced and controlled by the dominating gland. This dominance of one particular gland over the others is built into the genetic structure and has a significant impact on the metabolic processes in the body. These metabolic processes take up raw materials such as carbohydrates, fats, proteins in different proportions and occur in the presence of catalysts that are available through micronutrients such as minerals and vitamins. The difference in proportions of raw material utilized is due to the functioning differences between these glands of the endocrine system. The classification is

done into 4 main categories – adrenal (controls reaction to environmental stresses and dangers), gonad (controls reproduction and growth), thyroid (controls metabolism) and pituitary (control the secretion of all glands) depending upon the dominating gland. Different diets and exercise routines are recommended for different body types.

3. The third classification technique and most commonly used in the context of weight management programs is on the basis of Somatotype. The system is based on identifying the association between psychological behavior patterns or temperament with the body structure of the individual. Under this system it is believed that the characteristic behavioral patterns as exhibited by an individual are typical of his or her own body type to a significantly large extent. The body type as in other classification systems is genetically predetermined. People having a similar body type are expected to show similar behavioral traits under this system. The system of classification is on the basis of the 3 elements or Somatotypes that are named after cell groups known as *germinal epithelium* formed during the growth of the embryo in the womb. The three Somatotypes are named after the three germ layers - *mesoderm, endoderm* and *ectoderm* and are therefore called Mesomorph, Endomorph and Ectomorph respectively. Mesomorphs are characterized by a predominance of lean muscle, connective tissues and bone; Endomorphs are characterized by a predominant roundness & softness in the different parts of the body as a consequence of excess body fat; Ectomorphs are characterized by fragility & linearity and are therefore possess frail and weak body structures which are devoid of fat as well as lean muscle. An individual may not necessarily be a pure Somatotype and can be a combination of one or more of these Somatotypes.

These body types are not inflexible to change arising from application of stimulus in the form of exercise and diet. Not each and every one possesses a dream body shape and structure by birth. Similarly, not everyone who has the nature predisposition to a good physique is able to maintain it. The genetic code embedded into our body in the form of body type plays a significant role in determining our body shape but it is not the only parameter. It is true that an Ectomorph may ingest large number of calories as part of diet and may perform rigorous strength training routines but still may find it difficult to add an extra pound of weight. Similarly, an endomorph may perform long duration cardiovascular workouts but still may not be able to shed those extra pounds of fat stored in the body. However, genetic predisposition only indicates the difficulty to create changes; nowhere does it mention that it is impossible. Moreover, in most cases an individual is a combination of Somatotypes which makes it possible to create changes in one direction or the other depending upon the requirement. It is therefore of utmost importance to identify the body type and the goals before designing an exercise program and diet plan. Once this identification has been done, adherence to a scientifically designed weight management program will lead to achievement of the desired targets that have been set.

Components of Weight Management Program

A healthy weight management program should be based on the four pillars of wellness – physical fitness, balanced diet & nutrition, rest & relaxation and mental attitude. A balance between all the four components is crucial for the success of a weight management program. A good fitness routine which is not accompanied by an appropriate diet will not help the individual trying to lose weight. Similarly, a person who does not have the right mental frame of mind will find it extremely difficult to adhere to certain basic restrictions that such a program may impose; as a result of which the whole program fails. A weight management program needs to be customized according the needs and goals of the individual. This customization needs to be reflected in all the components as well. In case even one of them is not in sync it can derail the whole program itself.

Balanced Diet & Nutrition

A good balanced and nutritious diet is paramount to the success of a weight management program. Not only should it provide the right amount of energy depending upon the goals of the program, it should also provide the necessary micronutrients in adequate quantities for long term sustainable weight loss and overall health. A balanced diet incorporates energy compounds such as carbohydrates, fats and proteins, micronutrients such as vitamins and minerals as well as fiber and water in adequate quantities. As mentioned before the quantity and proportion of the main energy compounds depends on the goal of the program while micronutrients should be available to the body as per standard guidelines such as DV (Daily Value), RDA (Recommended Dietary Allowance) and EAR (Estimated Average Requirement).

In case the goal is to lose weight then an energy deficit needs to be created in a way that energy intake is less than energy output. This may involve reducing the quantities of the energy compounds from the normal diet and vice versa in case weight gain is the goal. As part of a weight management diet plan identifying the calorie content of meals is extremely crucial. To lose one pound of fat, a deficit of 3,500 calories needs to be created. This can be done by ensuring a regular deficit of 500 calories per day throughout the week. A gradual weight loss rate of one to two pounds per week is ideal for the body since it gets time to adapt to the changed conditions. Moreover, gradual weight loss ensures that there is least amount of muscle loss that happens as part of the weight loss process. This is where the efficacy of crash diets or very low calorie diets is questioned. Apart from loss of muscle tissue they cause micronutrient deficiency extremely dangerous to overall health. Certain research studies also confirm that such diets in fact may lead to fat gain since the body experiences starvation and tends to preserve the energy dense compounds for later utilization. This is done at the expense of lean muscle tissue which is difficult to maintain in the body.

In general any meal should include around 55 to 60% energy being provided through carbohydrates, 25 to 30% energy through fats and approximately 10 to 20% through proteins. This principally ensures that while all the energy requirements are met, nourishment of the body is not compromised upon. Even in case an energy deficit is required for losing weight it created in such a way that all nutrients including fats are available to the body for essential functions that need to be performed for healthy a mind & body.

Once the energy requirements have been calculated the next step in the preparation of a balanced diet plan is identification of the meals and meal content. By identification of the meals, it is intended to finalize the meal frequency and the meal timings such that they can be incorporated in the lifestyle in an easy manner. Too many alteration in the existing pattern of life make the adherence to the plan that much more difficult. Therefore, a diet plan should be designed taking into consideration the individual's lifestyle and preferences. In this context the question of meal frequency becomes a pertinent one. The three meal plan has been ingrained into modern day diets since it is conveniently adopted into work life pattern. It may not necessarily be as good and efficient for overall health as well as for weight loss in comparison to a high frequency diet plan such as a 6 meal plan.

Our body requires energy at a particular rate; this rate is defined by our metabolic rate but there may be spikes in demand such as the post exercise period. Clearly, the body does not require energy at the rate at which we eat and the rate at which the energy is released in our body upon digestion of food. In such a situation the excess energy needs to be stored in the body to be utilized at a later stage. The body can do it in the form of glycogen in the liver and muscles but once these limited space stores are filled up then it converts the extra energy into fat which can be stored all over the body. Secondly, whenever a heavy meal is consumed the insulin spike that occurs upon increase in glucose level in the blood, stays on for a longer period of time. In a similar manner this also results in storage of carbohydrates initially as glycogen but later on as fat. Smaller meals ensure that the body gets energy at a rate commensurate to its requirements so that it does not have to convert and store it as body fat. A high frequency 6 meal plan aids in this process of immediate utilization.

The other factor is the proportion of energy that is derived from stored energy reserves versus that derived from food that has been consume in the recent past. The body stores energy compounds like glucose in the blood, glycogen or long chain glucose molecules in the liver and muscles. And fat in the adipose tissue. Whenever the requirement for energy arises the body meets it through one of these sources. When extra carbohydrates are ingested as part of the meal the body stops utilizing the fat stored in the body, on top of this, the extra carbohydrate gets converted into fat. In a high frequency meal plan, the amount of carbohydrates consumed in any meal is limited, which prevents prolonged insulin spike from occurring. This helps in preventing conversion of carbohydrates into fat and also helps in utilizing stored fat for meeting energy requirement.

As part of weight management programs high frequency smaller meals are often suggested due to the aforementioned reasons. The other psychological advantages offered by these plans are beneficial in ensuring adherence during the initial difficult periods of change. By trimming down meal quantities and increasing frequency, cravings that lead to unplanned eating can be prevented. Since, as part of the meal itself there are many meals, the meal content is pre-planned and hence, the chances of eating something unhealthy out of the diet plan are reduce. Uncontrolled hunger pangs are also not experienced since the gap between meals is shorter. This has a dual advantage – apart from preventing binge eating it also helps in avoiding overeating during the main meals. The effect of frequent meals on metabolism has also been seen to be positive in nature. By eating frequent meals, the body is not allowed to go onto starvation mode and thereby the metabolism is maintained at a high since there it is made to experience a near constant availability of food and energy. Increased metabolism helps in burning the extra fat reserves in the body and hence helps in losing weight in a desirable manner. In summary, a high frequency smaller meal plan seems to be much more effective in reducing body fat percentage in comparison to the modern day three meal plan. This loss in fat percentage is ideal for weight loss as well as weight gain. Hence such a meal plan can be made an integral part of any weight management program.

Physical Exercise As Part of Weight Management Plan

The second pillar in a healthy weight management program is regular physical exercise at the right intensity. It helps in increasing the energy output to create the deficit that is essential for weight loss to take place. In case weight gain is the goal, exercise provides stimulus forcing the body to grow to meet the additional demands placed on it. Whatever the goals may be, like a healthy weight management plan, a healthy exercise routine should include all the components – cardiovascular endurance, muscular endurance, muscular strength and flexibility.

1. Cardiovascular endurance exercises include all those exercises that involve repetitive movement of large muscle groups at a heart rate greater than resting heart rate.

Exercises include running, jogging, swimming, cycling, rowing etc. The role of the cardiovascular system is to ensure efficient delivery of oxygen to different parts of the body. Performing regular cardio exercises not only improves the delivery mechanism of oxygen but also helps improve the efficiency of the vascular system and the exercising muscles to take up and utilize the oxygen delivered. Chronic adaptations as a result of cardio activities help in preventing cardiovascular and coronary artery diseases, metabolic disorders such as diabetes and metabolic syndrome and may also help in preventing certain forms of cancer.

2. Muscular endurance exercises help improve the endurance of different muscle groups in the body. Numerous activities of daily life involve repeated movements to be performed of a particular type and therefore utilize a particular muscle group. Improved muscular endurance helps in performing these movements without experiencing too much fatigue in the exercising muscle.

3. Muscular strength is the ability of a particular muscle to lift heavy loads. In daily life, the requirement to lift and carry heavy load often arises but infrequently. If the body is deconditioned to perform such a movement then there is risk of injury. Strength training exercises help in increasing lean muscle tissue in the body as well as improves the quality of bone health by strengthening them. In such a manner it helps in performing activities of daily life.

4. Flexibility refers to pain free range of motion around a joint. This is one of the most neglected aspects of fitness and as age progresses it becomes the most important component. Flexibility training in the form of static stretches held for moderate to long durations helps in improving flexibility which then reduced the risk of injuries.

All these components of exercise are important in the context of weight management but more emphasis is directed towards exercises such as cardiovascular workouts. These exercises increase the heart rate in such a manner that the extra demands placed on the body force it to rely on stored energy reserves in the body. By careful planning of diet and intensity of workout it is possible to selectively utilize fat stored in the body for meeting the energy requirements. A balanced routine should include 40 minutes of moderate intensity aerobic activity for 3 to 4 times a week, strength training or resistance training of all the muscle groups at least twice a week and static stretching to improve flexibility should also be incorporated at least 2 to 3 times a week. Such a balanced workout leads to weight loss as well as improves overall physical fitness.

Rest & Relaxation

It is important to understand that the actual growth and development of the body does not take place while exercise is being performed. Exercise only provides the stimulus required for growth and development of tissues. The other ingredients that ensure that the purpose is fulfilled are balanced & nutritious diet and rest & relaxation. Post exercise when the body rests and is provided energy and nutrition is the time when the actual growth happens. At this stage the energy requirements should be met from within the fat stores for weight loss to take place. In case this is not done, the body will strip lean muscle tissue to meet the demands post by exercise. Also, in case enough rest is not provided to the body, the chance of overtraining leading to injury increases manifold. Adequate amount of rest and relaxation also helps in maintaining hormonal balance in the body. This is also crucial for healthy weight management.

Mental Attitude

A perfectly designed diet plan or a perfectly designed exercise routine is of no use if the individual for whom it is designed is not able to adhere to it. This is where the role of a positive mental attitude comes into picture. Psychological factors play an important role in weight management than is generally imagined. In fact adherence to any plan is solely dependent on the attitude a person carries towards the lifestyle alteration that is being imposed as part of the plan. In case the weight management program is looked at as a set of limitations or restrictions that is forced, the chances of adherence in the short run as well as over a period of time diminish significantly. On the contrary an individual adopting a positive attitude looks at the program as a new positive lifestyle which is embraced with vigour and excitement.

Yoga for Weight Management

'Yoga' is derived from '*yuj*' in Sanskrit which means 'to unite'. Originating in ancient India, it is a unique combination of mental, physical as well as spiritual disciplines. This union that yoga refers to is the union of the individual with the universal. Yoga is believed to have originated more than 25,000 years ago and contrary to common knowledge it is not just a sequence of poses and postures for improving health and fitness. It is an ancient science that includes tools such as *pranayama* or breathing methods and techniques, meditation also called *dhyana* and finally physical postures or *asanas*.

The modern form of yoga is believed to have begun with Parliament of Religions convened in Chicago in the year 1893. In the convention *Swami Vivekanand* had a deep impact on the thinking of the audience. In subsequent tours in the United States he promoted various aspects of yoga. These talks and lectures led to yoga shedding the tag of a purely religious practice and being accepted by the western world. In the years since then health benefits emanating through regular yogic practices have been researched, documented and published all over the world. It is estimated that in the US alone more than 25 million people practice yoga on a regular basis.

The myriad benefits of yoga include physiological benefits such as improved flexibility, increased strength, better posture, weight loss, effective breathing, stronger immune system, improved bone strength and improvement in medical conditions such as migraine and insomnia; psychological benefits include stress relief, greater awareness, improved energy levels and an overall feeling of inner peace. Yoga is quite efficient in weight loss as well. It advocates a multi dimensional approach that incorporates physical, emotional and spiritual components and does not superficially work on eliminating the symptoms alone. The root cause of the problem is targeted through yoga to deal with the weight problem. It therefore involves detoxification, increasing metabolism, achieving hormonal balance, improving observation & awareness and cardiovascular endurance.

Certain forms of yoga prescribe movements done at a rapid pace in a sequential manner that elevates heart rate to moderate or high levels and in such a manner mimic cardiovascular activities. This is very similar to circuit training which is a form of strength training where each muscle group is exercises one after the other without any rest. Such workout principles help in weight loss since heart rate is maintained at a moderate to high level for considerable duration. Apart from the *asanas* that are practiced, *kriyas* such as *kapalbhati* done at a vigorous intensity provides a good cardiovascular endurance workout. Different *asanas* also have different effects on the mind as well. Certain movements performed at a particular pace are known to provide calmness, while other movements help in boosting energy levels. Yoga *asanas* also improve thyroid and pituitary health and balanced secretion of hormones helps in improving metabolism to suit the body's requirements. Other benefits such as reduction in anxiety and detoxification of the body indirectly help in losing weight in a healthy manner. The psychological benefits such as improved awareness and sense of calmness help in immensely improving adherence to weight management program since they bring about a positive attitude towards the entire process.

Meditation for Weight Management

Meditation refers to the process of reflection and contemplation that helps in calming the mind and in this way relieves stress and anxiety. It has been commonly linked with religion and prayer across many cultures since ancient times. It is often thought of as a tool to improve concentration and as an aid to attaining peace of mind, a path to God and spirituality. Meditation is commonly done by mental exercises that include concentrated breathing, single point focussing as well as chanting. In some cultures it is performed by being completely detached from external worldly contacts while in others the person may interact with the outside world while practicing meditation.

Meditation has developed over centuries and across cultures and civilizations. There is no one form of meditation that fits all the requirements and is ideal for each and everyone practicing it. Which form suits whom depend on factors like state of mind, personality traits and external surroundings. The meditation form that should be practiced is the one in which the person feels most comfortable rather than going after something which is perceived by people in close contact to be most helpful. There is no one single source or authority or text that is referred to for meditation practices. Numerous different forms have evolved over ages each having certain distinct characteristics. A high proportion of these forms though, involve awareness of breath as the underlying platform on which meditation is practiced. Different types of meditation include the following:

1. *Mindfulness meditation* is a popular practice in the West in which awareness of the surroundings is not blocked out. The idea in this practice is to allow all the thoughts to flow into the mind without focusing on any single one of them. This form does not necessarily require quiet and peaceful surroundings and can be performed anywhere. Breathing like most meditation forms is important but is not the primary and sole element. It is a form which is suited to beginners who may find concentrating and blocking out thoughts to focus on nothingness extremely difficult.
2. *Focused meditation* involves focusing on a single thought throughout the practice session. The point of focus can be internal like an imagined object and can also be external in nature like a chant. The emphasis is not on the thought but on the process of maintaining concentration and not losing focus.
3. *Spiritual meditation* is a form which is closely interlinked with religion and is suited to individuals who offer prayers as part of their daily rituals. The emphasis is on communication and interaction with God and union with the Universal.
4. *Trance based meditation* is an advanced form of spiritual meditation that involves reaching a state of trance by losing self control induced by usage of intoxicating substances. Since the person practicing this form of meditation may not have any memory of the experience, it has a very limited usage, if any, on daily life.
5. *Movement meditation* is a form in which the practice involves constant movement. These movements can be slow & rhythmic in nature such as swaying of the body. These gentle movements are believed to have a calming influence on the mind.
6. *Other forms of meditation* include mantra meditation, transcendental meditation, *kundalini* meditation, *Qi gong*

meditation and *Zazen* meditation. Each of them originating in different ages and different parts of the world; differing in the way they are practiced and in terms of their end objectives as well.

Since it is not an exact science, the benefits of meditation cannot be directly and objectively measured. Interest in the scientific community has increased immensely as a result of observations, but studies and research has not determined conclusive proof of benefits derived from meditation. Physical benefits include elimination of stress leading to improvement in conditions such as hypertension and diabetes. The vibrations released are also known to have the added effect of diminishing the negative impact of the disease. Meditation is known to reduce the level of Cortisol and hence reduces stress levels; it also reduces the accumulation of lactic acid which is associated with anxiety. Meditation helps in breath control thereby reducing heart rate and helping the body fight against hypertension; it helps to improve immunity, provides balance to the hormonal system, improves fertility, reduces cholesterol level and helps in weight loss.

While weight loss cannot be directly achieved through meditation it has a more important role to play than any other parameter including physical exercise and diet & nutrition. Meditation does not burn fat in the body but it provides a frame of mind and attitude that is crucial for the efficient functioning of the tools that result in weight loss. Without a positive frame of mind adherence to the weight management program is practically impossible. Meditation helps in identifying the root cause of the weight problem and it does not superficially work on the symptoms of the problem. Even if an individual on a weight loss program is able to achieve weight loss, it may not be sustainable and permanent in case the root cause is not tackled. Meditation helps in improving self control and thereby increases determination that helps in adhering to the program. Moreover, the positive attitude with which the program is adopted magnifies the benefits that may be derived. From the psychological perspective of filling in voids, people have a tendency to go on binges – commonly termed as emotional eating. Meditation helps by working on elimination of desire itself helping the individual practicing it to remain unaffected by the pressures of daily home and work life. The positive attitude that is manifested helps to attain a balance in life. This balance prevents excessive emotions either positive or negative. The person thus practicing experiences an ever prevalent calmness irrespective of the external environment and the alterations that these parameters may undergo. While meditation objectively may not lead to weight loss in the conventional sense, it empowers the individual with a positive attitude – the most useful tool in attaining any weight loss goal.

Meditation also provides numerous psychological benefits. It helps ease stress & anxiety as mentioned earlier. A person becomes calm & composed and is able to visualize the external world with detachment helping in decision making process. Meditation also recharges and provides a feeling of rejuvenation which increases efficiency of all work that the person indulges in. Practicing meditation on a regular basis provides greater mental control that helps in curbing fluctuations in mood and emotion. The spiritual benefits that are derived from regular practice of meditation are manifested in the attitude of kindness and compassion towards others. Union of mind, body and soul leads to an infinite source of love. All these benefits from meditation practice helps produce a balanced personality unfazed by external events and conditions.

Conclusion

For a successful weight management program it is imperative that all these components or pillars be incorporated. When these pillars are not in sync the chances of success of these plans reduces considerably. In fact, neglecting any one of these components may compromise short term as well as long term health and wellness. On the other hand when the wavelengths of the efforts do not match it is very unlikely that the weight management goals are achieved. A positive attitude towards a weight management program that includes a well rounded physical fitness routine, a balanced diet & nutrition plan and sufficient rest & relaxation is almost a guarantee to achieving long term and sustainable weight loss.

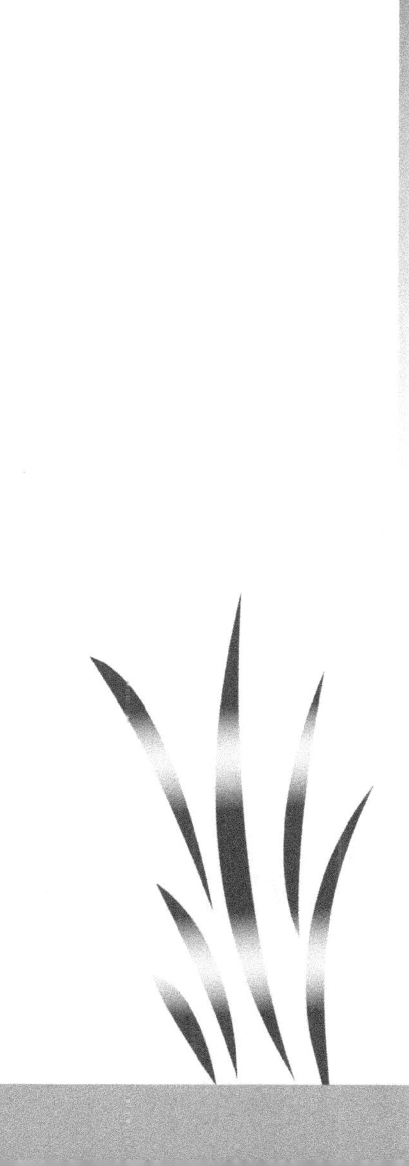

Goals

Goals

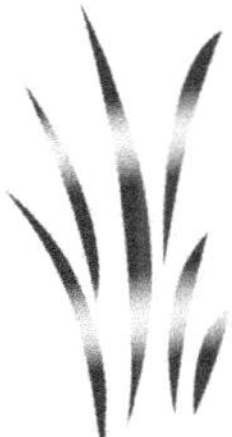

Body Type

Body type also known as constitution type refers to the various methods of classifying the human body into distinct categories. The systems have either a theoretical or an empirical base. These classification systems help to a certain extent in grouping individuals and prescribing medical, exercise and nutritional programs. Some of these classification systems use body shape as the parameter to segregate different body types into respective categories. Body shapes are generally defined by the skeletal structure of the individual. It also depends upon the amount of lean muscle tissue and fat distributed over the body. The skeletal or bone framework of an individual starts growing at the embryo stage itself even before birth and continues till adulthood, after which this growth comes to a halt. It then remains more or less the same for the remaining lifetime of the individual.

Different Classification Methodologies

Much before the concepts of genetic inheritance came into the forefront, physicians practicing the science of *Ayurveda* in ancient India recognized the fact that these inherited genetic traits are seen in groups. For example, in the current context, an Indian skin color is not expected to be matched with blue eyes of the individual. Similarly, in case genetically a person has a strong muscular build, it is bound to happen that this person shall have a heavy bone structure as well as strong connective tissues to support the musculature. Unlike the first example this is simpler to identify the logical connect in this case. The *Ayurvedic* physicians understood this grouping pattern and developed a medical system which takes into consideration this very understanding.

No one particular exercise routine or weight management plan or even lifestyle pattern can be ideal for everyone. Over thousands of generations we have adapted according to the requirements posed by the environment around us. We have been able to survive by evolving in this particular manner, changing slowly but surely in infinitesimally small steps. Each step is encoded into our DNA. It is the historical account of our evolution. By understanding our genetic type we will be able to understand what works best for us.

Over years of hard work, researchers have been able to develop different classification systems to identify and pin point the common differences between groups of people. Each classification system has a basis for doing so. The initial systems focused on religion, time of birth, race & class as the basis of differentiation. Methods such as sex, blood type, anatomical structure gradually came to be accepted in the next stage of evolution of this study. Most methods of classification may have some or the other form of authenticity, but research scientists over the years have zeroed in upon three methods to make this classification – anatomical, energy and glandular. There is also a definite purpose as to why any of this system does this classification. The purpose may be for understanding the psychology or temperament and categorizing individuals or it may be for the purpose of forming a weight management diet & exercise routine. Each system believes in compartmentalizing according to some basic parameter, although within the category too, catering to individual differences is imperative.

Glandular or Metabolic Types

In the glandular or metabolic method, classification of people is done into various groups on the basis of the gland that is dominant in the endocrine system. Under this system it is believed that in each person the biochemical reactions happening are influenced considerably by the dominant gland. This dominance of one particular gland over others is something that is built into our genetic structure and has an effect on numerous metabolic and biochemical activities happening continuously in our body.

Metabolism is the process by which our body is able to utilize all the raw material that it consumes and convert it into energy and other building blocks essential for the sustenance of life. These raw materials include energy compounds such as carbohydrate, protein and fat, micro nutrients such as vitamins & minerals, as well as air and water. During the continuous metabolic processes happening in the cells of our body these different raw materials are taken up in different proportions indifferent individuals. Some individuals may require more of one particular raw material such as carbohydrates while others may require more of proteins. This difference is created due to the differences in the functioning of the different glands. The 4 glands of the endocrine system that form the basis of this classification methodology are:

1. Adrenal gland controls our reaction to environmental dangers and stresses
2. Gonad controls growth and reproduction
3. Thyroid gland determines the rate at which energy is utilized and the metabolic rate
4. Pituitary gland is the master key and controls the secretion of all the other glands

Certain exercises and foods can stimulate as well as inhibit the secretion and activity of one or more of these glands. Cravings are generally satiated first by individuals and this is what stimulates the dominant gland most. The secretion from this dominant gland affects the brain and manipulates the balance of the body. In case the cravings are repeatedly fulfilled, the dominant gland is over stimulated, leading to imbalance and exhaustion. It may even lead to the gland stopping to function in an appropriate manner. Similarly, in case a particular gland is under stimulated then activities related to that gland may become less prominent. Overall, in both cases an imbalance is created. This imbalance is manifested as physical as well as emotional disturbances. As mentioned earlier, the key to this system is to restore the balance of the body so that all the glands are functioning in a synchronized manner. To restore this balance a balanced exercise program and a healthy diet have been prescribed as part of the system. One has to cut out the cravings and feed on food stuff that stimulates the other glands of the body. Gradually the chemical balance that had been thwarted is restored. Eventually this leads to greater energy levels in the individual and lesser amounts of stress experienced.

Determining the glandular type is done by analyzing parameters such as anatomical characteristics – body shape, skeletal structure, body fat distribution pattern as well as the response that the body gives upon eating certain food types such as energy rich compounds like glucose.

This methodology divides all individuals in to one of 4 main groups as explained above, and each of these groups have certain characteristic traits in terms of physical appearance, diet preference and behavioral pattern.

Adrenal

The adrenal glands are responsible for development of lean muscle tissue & storage of fat; they also control the energy systems within the body along with stimulating appetite. All in all, they help to maintain a balance in the body. The person whose adrenal gland dominates is physically seen to be strong and have a well developed skeletal structure emphasized by broad shoulders and wide chest. They have a strong muscular structure with some amount of fat in the torso, and a large square shaped head. To carry this heavy structure legs are also very strong specifically the larger muscle groups such as quadriceps and hamstrings. Women generally have larger breasts in comparison to other groups and men and women both have buttocks which are generally flatter.

These individuals are stable as well as consistent. They have a clear understanding of what they want and there is significant hunger for power and being in control. This is certainly visible in their healthy appetite and pretty strong dietary preferences. They crave for foods that stimulate adrenal glands include meat, chicken, cheese and eggs. They are attracted towards food that is full of flavor and is rich in content. Since people in this group are prone to putting on weight especially in the abdominal region, the problem with such an attraction is that these foods not only increase the fat percentage in the body but also lead to hypertension, insomnia, constipation, gout and other stress induced issues. People in this category also have a tendency to store toxins in the colon as well as in the muscles which then leads to body pains, as well as digestive issues such as bloating and gas formation.

Individuals in this group should choose new foods that stimulate the other glands as well, so that an appropriate balance is created. A vegetarian diet is ideal for these people, though it may be close to impossible to give up the adrenal stimulating foods altogether. However, characteristically these people have strong will power and are able to achieve what they set their minds to. Ideally breakfast should not be a very heavy meal and can comprise of cereal, lunch again should be light with lots of greens and some protein, supper can be the heaviest meal of the day and higher protein content in the meal will also ensure that post supper they are able to sleep well. As part of general dietary guidelines people in this group should take care of the following points:

Individuals in this group may find exercises such as playing tennis really interesting and stimulating. The goal should be accumulate some amount of cardiovascular workout and flexibility exercises during the day. Resistance training especially heavy weight lifting is not recommended for such people because of already raised energy levels and that these activities may create a greater imbalance.

Gonad

This particular body type is pertinent only to women. The individuals that belong to this category are very feministic in nature. They have a characteristic pear shaped physique with extra wide hips and thighs with very narrow shoulders. When women become overweight they tend to carry a lot of fat on the outer thighs which can be very difficult to get rid of. Characteristically women in this category are peace loving, warm and nurturing. In general it has been experienced that women with this body type are not pro competition but may actually stand up for anything that they strongly believe in.

The types of food that attract people in this group are creamy as well as spicy foods that stimulate the gonad or sex glands. The rich food leads to accumulation of fat, but this takes place at a slightly slower rate. They find it difficult to break down fat molecules in food and this leads to quite a bit of imbalance. Fatigue and nausea are often experienced after a heavy meal. They are prone to issues such as arthritis, allergies, kidney and gall bladder problems, and issues with female sex organs. These issues come about since the body is not able to break the fat down and it gets stored as toxins within the system. People in this group should therefore avoid fried foods such as chips, spices, sugar, cream, organ meat and caffeine.

Breakfast should be light and can include fruits along with a little lean protein source. Lunch should consist of fresh salads without any creamy dressings. The dominant sex glands as can be expected are active during the night and this when the largest protein meal should be consumed. However, care needs to be taken that the meal is not very heavy otherwise sleep gets disturbed for people in this group. A general rule that is even more pertinent in case of this group is that enough water should be consumed between the meals.

The exercises that can be taken up include cardiovascular activities such as running and jogging, as well as aerobic activities that work on the lower body. Activities such as gymnastics are also recommended for this group since they tend to work on creating a balance between the lower and upper halves of the body, which is an issue that this group faces.

Pituitary

Individuals in this category are generally considered soft, with distributed baby fat all over the body. Females generally have smaller hips and breasts. Males in this group seem to possess large heads in comparison to the rest of the body framework. Characteristically, individuals in this group are the least physical in nature. Individuals in this category are the ones who did not develop physically at a pace at which others did. They appear lost and dreamy and enjoy activities that stimulate the mind. These include the philosophers and researchers who can produce dramatic pieces of work if given an opportunity to work without much disturbance.

The digestive system is generally weak and therefore cravings are for foods that are light such as milk, yogurt and cheese. Apart from a particular liking for these foods, there is an attraction for other foods such as simple & complex carbohydrates. Eating of dairy products as mentioned before, stimulates the pituitary gland. Over stimulation can lead to allergies, gastrointestinal & colon related problems and skin conditions. People in this group also do not reach physical maturity fast and may also face many sex related problems, this is a direct result of issues with the pituitary gland. To create balance, in case a dietary change is required such as substituting dairy products with other foods, this group finds it the easiest to incorporate such a change. Increasing the protein intake as part of the diet is also extremely crucial. This protein should essentially come from non-dairy sources only. People in this group should try and consume a heavy breakfast as well as a heavy lunch while keeping the dinner light. All three meals should incorporate a high percentage of protein from a variety of sources other than dairy products.

Activities such as martial arts, yoga, tai chi and dance are recommended. Regular activities such as walking become monotonous and people in this group tend to think of other things while performing these mechanical movements. It is therefore preferred that an activity that requires a higher level of concentration is chosen to be performed on a regular basis.

Thyroid

The Thyroid gland is responsible for ensuring a stable metabolic rate in the body. The physical characteristics of individuals in this group include wide shoulders and narrow hips which is characteristically a swimmer's physique. They have a tendency to add on fat around the chest and torso. Thyroid glands are very erratic in nature, and therefore the people in whom this is the dominating gland naturally have numerous mood fluctuations. They can exhibit immense lethargy at one point in time and at another they could be bursting with energy with the aim to produce something creative. Professions such as art & music are suitable for such individuals with high latent capacity for quality creative work.

Stimulating food for thyroid gland include simple sugars as well as complex carbohydrates. As is expected craving and satiation leads to overstimulation of the thyroid glands causing numerous issues. It is therefore best for people in this group to avoid foods such as white flour, sugar, fruit juices, bread, pasta and fried carbohydrates such as wafers and chips. Ideal replacements are foods that are high in protein such as lean meats such as chicken, fish and eggs. Caffeine should be replaced by green teas.

Exercises such as swimming as well as aerobic activities that are low impact in nature performed at least 3 times a week seem to be ideally suited to people in this group. Strenuous exercises that increase the heart rate over a certain level and maintain it there, are also not recommended since fatigue, exhaustion and energy swings are extremely common within this group. The intensity can be increased gradually once adherence to the exercise program is not under question.

It is important to understand that the glandular type or metabolic type of the body determines the ideal ratio in which macro nutrients should be consumed in the food. The theory clearly explains the reason for cravings and the need to curb the cravings. Over stimulating as well as under stimulating of the certain glands in the body creates an imbalance which then leads to health disorders. It is therefore important to correct this imbalance as soon as possible. This can be done through a properly designed exercise and diet program.

Energy Types

Classification on the basis of energy type is the oldest classification technique based on the ancient science of *Ayurveda* that originated in India. The classification is done on the basis of energy patterns, also called *doshas.* In *Ayurveda* it is believed that physical matter itself is largely made up of nothing with energy waves. The duality of particle and wave is understood by modern science today and the interaction between physical matter and energy waves was exactly the basis on which *Ayurveda* was practiced even in those ancient times. The field of medicine on the current date is beginning to study the interactions that exist between the endocrine system, central and peripheral nervous system and the immune system. The mode in which this communication takes place between the systems is not very clear but is evident that chemicals such as neuro-transmitters are utilized by the brain which is a part of the central nervous system, to do this communication.

In *ayurveda*, the universe is composed of five fundamental elements – *akasha* or space, *vayu* or air, *agni* or fire, *apu* or water *and prithvi* or earth. It is believed that human physiology like the universe is also composed of these five elements. The three *doshas* or biological humors are called *vata, pitta* and *kapha*. Each of them is a combination of two elements from the set of five constituent elements of the universe. *Vata or wind* is a combination of air and space, *pitta or bile* is a combination of water and fire and finally *kapha or phlegm* is a combination of earth and water. *Vata* controls movement both in the mind and the body; *pitta* regulates metabolic activities and finally *kapha* which is responsible for the structure. Each of these *doshas* has its sub-types and the combination of these *doshas* that we inherit at birth is responsible for everything that happens within us. Together these 3 *doshas* achieve a state of harmony in all aspects of our life when they are present in equal quantities thus being able to create a balance. When this balance is disturbed it gets manifested in various unhealthy ways.

Each individual has the three *doshas* in a particular proportion. This is similar to being ingrained in our genetic code. This combination of *doshas* is said to be *prakriti* and is different for each individual. It is uncommon to have all three *doshas* in equal proportions; generally each individual will have a combination of 2 dominant *doshas* and one which is not. Specifically there are 10 possible combinations for the *prakriti* of an individual. These are as following:

1. *Vata – prakriti* in which *vata* is dominant over other two doshas
2. *Pitta – prakriti* in which *pitta* is dominant over other two doshas
3. *Kapha – prakriti* in which *kapha* is dominant over other two doshas
4. *Vata – Pitta – prakriti* in which *vata & pitta* are the two dominant *doshas* with *vata* overriding *pitta*
5. *Pitta – Vata – prakriti* in which *pitta & vata* are the two dominant *doshas* with *pitta* overriding *vata*
6. *Vata – Kapha – prakriti* in which *vata & kapha* are the two dominant *doshas* with *vata* overriding *kapha*
7. *Kapha – Vata – prakriti* in which *kapha & vata* are the two dominant *doshas* with *kapha* overriding *vata*
8. *Pitta – Kapha – prakriti* in which *pitta & kapha* are the two dominant *doshas* with *pitta* overriding *kapha*
9. *Kapha – Pitta – prakriti* in which *kapha & pitta* are the two dominant *doshas* with *kapha* overriding *pitta*
10. *Vata – Pitta – Kapha – prakriti* in which there is a balance between the three *doshas*

As was the case in glandular system of classification, in *ayurveda* too, all the three *doshas* influence each and every individual but one particular *dosha* may be dominant as described above. It is believed in *ayurveda* that all ailments arise as a result of imbalance that is created in the *doshas*. The first step therefore, in any *ayurvedic* treatment plan is to identify the *prakriti* of the person.

An *ayurvedic* physician does so by assessing the pulse of the person and understanding the imbalance in the body and the reason behind it. Only after this assessment, a treatment plan can be suggested to restore the balance.

By balance it needs to be clarified at this stage, it is meant that the original *prakriti* is maintained. This is essential for leading a good, healthy life. However, due to our lifestyle choices, dietary habits, choice of environment that we live in, nature of our relations with other people, a decrease or increase in one of the *doshas* may happen leading to movement away from *prakriti* and consequently causing an imbalance. It is because of this very reason that the aim of any *ayurvedic* treatment plan is always to restore the balance.

Vata Dosha

The characteristics of *vata dosha* include cool, lacking weight, dry, rough, tiny penetrating particles, moving continuously, unlimited and unbounded. Individuals with *vata* in their *prakriti* have a thin and wiry skeletal structure; have voluminous hair and skin that is dry. In terms of their behavior they are lively, quick in thought and action, are good speakers and are affable and therefore make friends easily. These individuals are extremely creative and their level of enthusiasm is generally very high. They sleep very light and prefer warmer climates.

Generally, people who have a dominant *vata* will exhibit the characteristics as mentioned above. However, issues arise when *vata* characteristics become aggravated beyond a certain level, creating an imbalance. Similarly, an imbalance is created when a person with *pitta* or *kapha* dominant *dosha* start exhibiting *vata* characteristics. This again is a sign of imbalance and needs to be corrected. The signs and symptoms that suggest a *vata* imbalance include constant tension and anxiousness, feeling of fatigue, restless sleep, dry and flaking skin, brittle hair with split ends, chapped lips and sore throat, indigestion, gas build up, limited attention span with tendency to keep on working and moving. The reasons for a *vata* imbalance can be consumption of extremely cold beverages, eating raw food, eating extremely dry food, exposure to cold conditions, travel exertions and increased stress levels.

Correction can be done through lifestyle changes such as following a *vata* balancing dietary routine as suggested by an *ayurvedic* physician. In *ayurveda* as a general practice, antidotes are generally exactly opposite to the problem. For example, to counter *vata* characteristic of dryness, include foods that are liquid in nature; to counter roughness, include soft foods; to counter the cold foods that are warm should be consumed. The following list includes tips on balancing *vata* through diet:

1. Food should be cooked and eaten when warm. Cooked cereals, vegetable soups and beverages such as almond milk should be consumed. Raw foods such as salads and sprouts should be avoided
2. Food should not be dry, therefore small quantities of clarified butter should be used for heating and olive oil should be used when needed as a dressing. Cooked foods such as grains and baked vegetables can be consumed. Dry foods such as cereals and crackers should be avoided
3. Foods that can be consumed include vegetables such as carrots, bottle gourd, beetroot and green leafy vegetables such as spinach; basmati rice and whole wheat Indian flat breads.
4. Nuts are good *vata* balancers. Almonds can be soaked at night and consumed in the morning. Other nuts such as cashews and walnuts can also be consumed.
5. Spices aide digestion and also have a warming effect. Combination of spices can be used for preparation of all dishes
6. A combination of salty, sour and sweet help in balancing *vata*. Therefore, all three tastes should be included as part of daily meal plan. Citrus fruits, dried fruit, salted nuts can be consumed. Bitter and pungent tasting foods should be avoided.
7. Warm water should be consumed at regular intervals throughout the day

The following list includes tips on lifestyle that help in balancing *vata:*

1. Meals should never be skipped. In fact the meals should also be consumed in a peaceful manner and not in a hurry while on the move.

2. *Vata dosha* is characterized by restlessness and continuous movement in an irregular and uncontrolled manner. The first shift should be towards a more manageable lifestyle routine with regular timings for most activities such as waking up, sleeping and eating.
3. Getting up early after adequate amount of rest and walking for at least 30 minutes on a daily basis helps in balancing *vata*
4. At least 30 minutes should be devoted to practice of meditation on a daily basis. It has a calming and soothing influence and helps in overcoming the restlessness that is so characteristic of a *vata* dominant individual
5. To take care of dry skin and to improve blood circulation an *ayurvedic* massage should be taken before shower or bath. Jojoba oil or almond oil can be used for the massage.
6. Body should be protected from the cold, and warm clothing should be worn whenever one moves outdoors.

Pitta Dosha

As mentioned in the previous section, *Pitta* is a combination water and fire. The characteristics of *pitta* include sharp, hot, burning, acidic, pungent, liquid, flowing in an uncontrolled manner. Individuals with *pitta* dominant *prakriti* have a medium sized skeletal structure, have thin hair with signs of thinning and premature graying and have a sensitive warm and fair skin. They are sharp and very determined in their approach towards things. They are extremely ambitious and have a purpose about everything that they do. Self confidence is extremely high and they also possess an entrepreneurial spirit. All these are typical signs of a *pitta* dominant *prakriti* of an individual.

Generally, people who have a dominant *pitta* will exhibit the characteristics as mentioned above. However, issues arise when *pitta* characteristics become aggravated beyond a certain level, creating an imbalance. Similarly, an imbalance is created when a person with *vata* or *kapha* dominant *dosha* start exhibiting *pitta* characteristics. This again is a sign of imbalance and needs to be corrected. The signs and symptoms that suggest a *pitta* imbalance include constant irritation and impatience, obsession with work, acidity and heartburn, sensitive skin, feeling warm and uncomfortable even when indoors, regular involvement in arguments, short temper and sarcasm as a part of speech.

As was the case with *vata,* restoration of balance can be done through lifestyle changes such as following a *pitta* balancing dietary routine as suggested by an *ayurvedic* physician. For example, to counter the liquid nature of *pitta*, include heavy foods that are dry in nature; to counter the heat foods that are cool should be consumed. The following list includes tips on balancing *pitta* through diet:

1. Foods that have a cooling effect are ideal for *pitta* balancing. These include fresh and juicy fruits such as pear, milk, almonds, dates and coconut
2. Foods that can be eaten include dry substances such as crackers, dry cereal, granola bars; vegetables such as carrots, asparagus, green leafy vegetables, cauliflower, broccoli and beans; basmati rice and whole wheat Indian flat breads. They are even better when consumed with *pitta* pacifying spices and chutneys. Other grains such as amaranth and oats can also be consumed.
3. Clarified butter should be utilized for cooking purposes since it is understood to cool both mind and body.
4. To aid in digestion buttermilk can be consumed along with meals and water consumed should be cool.
5. A combination of astringent, bitter and sweet help in balancing *pitta*. Therefore, all three tastes should be included as part of daily meal plan. Milk, soaked almonds, ripened fruits can be consumed. Salty and pungent tasting foods should be avoided.
6. Spices need to be chosen carefully so that they are not too hot and pungent. Spices such as turmeric, coriander, cumin, fennel and cinnamon can be consumed in small quantities.

The following list includes tips on lifestyle that help in balancing *pitta:*

1. To balance *pitta* one should first and foremost be cool, both emotionally and physically. Avoid getting out in the sun, on an empty stomach or even after having a sour or spicy meal.

2. At least 30 minutes should be devoted to practice of meditation on a daily basis. It helps to balance the emotions and helps to create harmony between mind, body and soul.
3. Since skin is sensitive, an *ayurvedic* massage would be immensely beneficial each day before a bath. For the purpose coconut oil should be used and a couple of drops of aromatic essential oils such as rose can be added.
4. No meal should be skipped. Breakfast and lunch should be relatively heavier in comparison to dinner which should be kept light. Skipping meals means there is a huge gap between two meals and that will result in acidity.
5. It is important to break the obsession that one has with work. A recreation activity should be an everyday affair, even though it may be for a small duration.
6. Protection from the sun and heat is important. In case one has to move out in the sun, wearing loose cotton clothing, using sun glasses and drinking plenty of water is imperative

Kapha Dosha

Kapha is a combination earth and water. The characteristics of *kapha* include sweet, stability, cold, soft, lubricating, unctuous and slippery. Individuals with *kapha* dominant *prakriti* have a large sized skeletal structure, thick & oily skin, wavy and thick set hair. They are extremely calm and stable, in speech as well as in thought. They are very loyal by nature and have a kind of serenity about them. They are heavy sleepers and feel very uncomfortable in clammy and wet environments. Their disposition is sweet and calm and a feeling of peace and comfort is experienced around them. All these are typical signs of a *kapha* dominant *prakriti* of an individual.

Generally, people who have a dominant *kapha* will exhibit the characteristics as mentioned above. However, issues arise when *kapha* characteristics become aggravated beyond a certain level, creating an imbalance. Similarly, an imbalance is created when a person with *vata* or *pitta* dominant *dosha* start exhibiting *kapha* characteristics. This again is a sign of imbalance and needs to be corrected. The signs and symptoms that suggest a *kapha* imbalance include easily gaining weight, fatigue and exhaustion despite no strenuous activity being performed, difficulty in waking up even after prolonged sleep, oily skin, oily hair, feeling of heaviness and congestion, slow digestion rate, lethargy and lack of motivation.

As was the case with *pitta,* restoration of balance can be done through lifestyle changes such as following a *kapha* balancing dietary routine as suggested by an *ayurvedic* physician. For example, to counter the oily nature of *kapha*, include foods that are dry in nature; to counter the heaviness, foods that are light but nourishing should be consumed; to counter the cold and sweet characteristics of *kapha* warm foods which have a tangy and spicy taste should be consumed. The following list includes tips on balancing *kapha* through diet:

1. Oily foods should be avoided. Clarified butter should be utilized for cooking purposes but only in very small quantities. Food should ideally be steamed or boiled along with spices heated in a little clarified butter for taste.
2. Light but foods that warm have a *kapha* balancing nature. These include vegetable soups, stews, dals, and combination of vegetables with some grains. Salt should be avoided, and as a substitute herbs and spices can be added for flavor.
3. A combination of astringent, bitter and pungent help in balancing *kapha*. Therefore, all three tastes should be included as part of daily diet. Apples, beans, cauliflower, broccoli are ideal. Sweet, sour and salty food dishes should be avoided as much as possible
4. Foods that can be eaten include dry substances such as low salt crackers, dry rice cakes; lighter grains such as millet and barley are ideal ; vegetables such as carrots, okra, asparagus, green leafy vegetables, cauliflower, broccoli and beans, green peppers and ginger should also be used since they have a favorable *kapha* balancing effect. They are even better when consumed with *kapha* pacifying spices.
5. To aid in digestion buttermilk can be consumed along with meals and plenty of warm water should be consumed, this aids in flushing out toxins from the body.
6. Spices should have a warming effect. These can include turmeric, coriander, cumin, fenugreek and cloves can be consumed in small quantities.

The following list includes tips on lifestyle that help in balancing *kapha:*

1. To balance *kapha* one should firstly start doing something. It could mean getting physical exercise for some duration every day; it could involve mental exercising such as solving puzzles and crosswords that challenge the mind. Meeting new people and building new relationships is an inherent *kapha* characteristic
2. No meal should be skipped and there should not be any fast. This is because *kapha* digestion and metabolism both tend to be slow. Breakfast should be light; lunch should be relatively heavier in comparison to dinner which should be kept light again.
3. High intensity activities are ideal for *kapha* balancing. This could include sports that have a high intensity interval kind of workout pattern such as squash and tennis. Endurance activities such as running can also be performed.
4. Oily skin should be cleaned daily and if possible even twice a day. This will eliminate the impurities and that get accumulated in skin pores due to oily nature of skin. Shampoo should be used for hair on alternate days for the same reason. An *ayurvedic* oil massage every day in the morning can help in removing toxins that are embedded in the pores and also help increase energy level
5. Protection from damp environment should be given importance. Warm spices can be used in water that should again be heated. Steam can be taken to open up blocked pores
6. At least 30 minutes should be devoted to practice of meditation on a daily basis. It helps to balance the emotions and helps to create harmony between mind, body and soul.
7. Due to imbalance, even after long sleep of more than 10 hours one may feel tired and exhausted, as if one has not slept at all. To improve the rest quality gradually, cut out sleep during the day and at night sleep early and get up before sunrise.

Although there is no direct relation between the energy and glandular systems, yet some equivalence may be established. *Vata dosha* corresponds to the thyroid type, *pitta dosha* corresponds to adrenal type and *kapha dosha* roughly correspond to gonad type. The energy type also corresponds to the response that is shown to sensory stimulation. By understanding the energy type it becomes possible to apply the holistic practice to achieve a state of harmonious balance between mind, body and soul.

Constitutional Psychology & Somatotype

In the 1940s, William Herbert Sheldon, an American psychologist developed the theory of constitutional psychology. The aim of this system was to identify the association between different body types with temperament and psychological behavior patterns of individuals. Within the context of this theory it was hypothesized that the physique or body structure of an individual has a direct correlation with the temperament or natural behavior pattern as exhibited. The body structure is genetically pre-determined and that causes people to exhibit typical personality traits coherent with those exhibited by people with similar body structures.

This theory is based on 3 basic elements also called Somatotypes. These have been named after groups of cells also called *germinal epithelium* which are formed during the process of growth of embryo into fetus. Also referred to as germ layers these are a pronounced presence in the vertebrates. These germ layers came to be known as *mesoderm, endoderm* and *ectoderm.*

Endoderm

Endoderm is a germ layer which is made up of flattened cells initially which then become columnar in nature. It forms a predominant portion of the epithelial lining of the lungs, trachea, pharynx and the digestive tube. Mainly it forms certain parts of the colon, pancreas, stomach, liver and the intestines – predominant portion of the digestive tract.

Ectoderm

Ectoderm is the beginning of the tissues that cover the surfaces of the body. It comes out first and is responsible for the formation of nerves, pigments, connective tissue heads, mammary glands, hair and most importantly the epidermis and the central nervous system.

Mesoderm

Mesoderm is the layer that is formed between the endoderm and ectoderm. It is responsible for the skeletal structure, urinary bladder, urethra, kidney and importantly the heart, skeletal muscles and blood vessels.

On the basis of the germ layers Sheldon laid down the framework for Somatotypes. Along with a team of associates numerous college students were photographed in the nude, from the front, rear and the side. The aim was to identify regularities in the different body types. After extensive observation and subsequent analysis, the three Somatotypes or extreme body structures were defined – endomorph, mesomorph and ectomorph.

Endomorphic structure was characterized by a predominant softness and roundness throughout different parts of the body. Mesomorphic structure was a predominance of bone, lean muscle and connective tissues. Ectomorphic structure was a symbolized by fragility and linearity. However, any body type was a combination of the three Somatotypes. The representation was done on a 7 point scale from 1 to 7 where 1 is the minimum and 7 is the maximum. Therefore, a person characterized by a pure endomorphic body type was represented as 7-1-1; a pure mesomorphic body type as 1-7-1 and a pure ectomorphic body type as 1-1-7. For example, 263 means 2 (low Endomorph), 6 (high Mesomorph) and 3 (low Ectomorph). In this way one body type can be compared with another body type. A basketball player will be around 147 while a good body builder will be a 173. It does not necessarily mean that all the traits are mixed together in the particular ratio. For example, 475 may mean a heavy build of Endomorph along with musculature of Mesomorph and height of the Ectomorph which may be above average. Once this had been done, on the basis of this number representation, individual characteristics and behavioral traits were predicted.

Within the structure of the research it was believed that a person with an endomorphic body will typically be contented, affable and would be able to share feelings easily. Mesomorphs would be aggressive, bold and adventurous while ectomorphs would typically be shy, introverted, inhibited and sensitive to pain. During this empirical study observers rated individuals on these characteristics and it was found that the correlation between the body type and the characteristic behavior did exist. There were quite a few questions that were raised on the method that was followed for the study. However, subsequent studies that eliminated the issues that were raised also came out with similar results. Despite the results shown by these studies, over the years, social learning researchers have refuted the results with counter arguments. According to them, learning plays an extremely important role in this link that is observed between body types and temperament and that there is no concrete direct correlation between the two. Each particular type of body is generally associated with particular characteristic traits, which have been stereotyped. This stereotype is further reinforced through different media such as marketing & advertising campaigns, movies, theatre etc. These stereotypes are then transmitted to children from adults who are exposed to these media. The children then learn and begin to incorporate these specific traits or characteristic behavior patterns as part of their natural demeanor. It is because of this reason that typical temperaments may be observed with a specific body type that an individual has.

Typical Characteristics of Somatotypes

The three main body types are – Endomorph, Mesomorph and Ectomorph. Each of these body types has specific characteristics some of them are alterable while some are not. The three body types can be modulated by body composition, which itself can be altered by specific weight management techniques. A person who is currently considered an endomorph may sometime in future begin to resemble an Ectomorph; while as age progresses a Mesomorph might begin to lose lean muscle tissue and begin to resemble an Endomorph.

Endomorph

Endomorphs are characterized by a large bone or skeletal structure and a wide waist and are usually referred to as being fat. They are predisposed to storing as well as retaining body fat. The following traits generally define an Endomorph:

- Pear shaped or round body
- Short and stocky with round head
- Wide shoulders and hips

- Wider front to back in comparison to measurements from side to side
- Lot of fat specially in the upper arms, core and thighs

Endomorphs have a tendency to gain weight very easily; however, a large portion is undesirable fat and not lean muscle. Their ability to compete in sporting activities that require an individual to be agile as well as weight bearing activities that are aerobic in nature such as running is severely restricted. Sporting activities that require pure muscular strength such as power lifting are perfect for an individual who has an endomorphic structure. Muscles especially of the upper legs – quadriceps and hamstrings are extremely strong. Along with this advantageous trait, their size is well suited, in fact ideal for sports such as rugby where bulk is crucial, provided it can be supplemented with enough power. Endomorphs also generally possess good lung capacity, making activities such as rowing suitable for them.

An endomorph should try and get rid of the excess body fat. Since their bodies are predisposed to gaining & storing a lot of fat, maintaining a healthy lifestyle is crucial. They should engage themselves in long duration, moderate intensity aerobic activity like biking and brisk walking. This will result in burning a number of calories on a daily basis, predominantly through oxidation of fat. Strength training should nevertheless be done to get a better muscle to fat ratio and thereby improving metabolism. Moderate weights at a fast training pace (extremely small rest periods between sets and exercises) should be employed while doing resistance training. Weight management system should primarily ensure a reduction in the intake of calories. It should contain frequent but small meals. By restricting the intake of simple carbohydrates and fats, a good weight management meal plan for an endomorph ensures that minimal amount of the intake is stored as body fat.

Mesomorph

Mesomorphs are characterized by wide shoulders, solid torso but narrow waist and are usually referred to as being muscular. They are invariably predisposed to increase in lean muscle tissue but not storing body fat. The following traits generally define an Mesomorph:

- Body is wedge shaped with a narrow waist
- Broad shoulders and cubical head
- Lean muscle tissue in arms and legs
- Narrow from front to back in comparison to measurement from side to side
- Low amount of stored body fat

A Mesomorph has a large and sturdy bone structure as well as higher mass of lean muscle, thereby providing a naturally athletic physique. Coupled with the tendency to gain lean muscle they excel in most sports because of physical characteristics such as muscular strength, speed and agility. These traits along with a good response to strength as well as cardiovascular training lay down a sound platform for body building as well. They are generally good at explosive kind of sports activities such as boxing and football.

Mesomorphs have a naturally fit body but proper exercise and diet as part of a weight management plan are essential towards maintaining this physique. Strength training should be done with moderate to heavy weights and for longer duration but with moderate rest periods between sets and exercises. Aerobic activities should be included in moderate amounts as a part of the exercise program. The metabolic rates of Mesomorphs are much faster than that of Endomorphs but slower than that of Ectomorphs. Since, Mesomorphs can gain some amount of fat slightly easily as compared to pure Ectomorphs, a good healthy weight management program is essential to maintain lean and muscular physique.

Ectomorph

Ectomorphs are characterized by long and thin limbs and are usually referred to as being slim. They are not predisposed to store fat or build muscle. The following traits generally define an Ectomorph:

- Thin arms & legs
- Hip and shoulders are narrow

- Chest & abdomen are narrow
- High forehead and a receding chin
- Little muscle or fat

An Ectomorph is generally slender and thin, and therefore strength and power activities & sports are not suitable for them. Lack of lean muscle tissue and consequently muscular strength puts them at a big disadvantage in sports activities that require mass. Their light frame makes them suited for long duration aerobic activities such as cycling & running as well as other activities such as gymnastics. Characteristic traits such as better thermo regulation provide them with an added advantage in endurance based sports.

It is possible that body fat in Ectomorphs drops to extremely low levels which can be dangerous to health and in case of females who participate in long duration endurance activities it can result in severe iron deficiency. Ectomorphs should concentrate on gaining weight in the form of good lean muscle tissue (some women who are too thin may also want to put on a little fat to look more feminine). Weight training should be done but not too often or for too long in each session. Workouts should be short and intense focusing on big muscle groups. Weights lifted should be moderately heavy and rest periods between sets should be longer for better recovery. Long duration aerobic activities should be kept to a minimum, to prevent undue loss of lean muscle tissue. They have an extremely fast metabolism which burns up calories very quickly. Therefore they need a huge amount of calories in order to gain weight. A high calorie diet is therefore required at the same time ensuring that low quality junk food is avoided.

Types of Body Shapes

Once we have a basic understanding of Somatotypes, we can move ahead and understand their practical application which essentially helps in defining body shape. The following is a list of different body shapes:

Male Ectomorphs

Male Ectomorphs are individuals with long and thin limbs – both arms and legs. Circumference of waist, ankle and wrist is very small. They do not gain weight and are called 'hard gainers' in common parlance. Even when they manage to gain some weight it is generally fat which is put in the abdominal region alone. They find it close to impossible to put on or gain any sort of lean muscle tissue. A big reason behind this is their extremely high metabolic rate. Despite these shortcomings, male ectomorphs are pretty good at long duration endurance activities such as biking and running.

Male Mesomorphs

Male Mesomorphs are muscular and are extremely athletic in nature. They generally have a large lean muscle mass base and this is clearly visible in their thick arms, wide chest, broad shoulders and strong legs & calves. They respond extremely well to exercise programs but in case of inactivity they tend to gain some weight also fast. It is therefore imperative the male Mesomorphs participate in regular physical activities to maintain their near perfect physiques.

Male Ecto–Mesomorphs

As the name of this body shape suggests, male ecto–mesomorphs are a combination of ectomorph and mesomorph somatotypes. Individuals in this category have a tendency to move between being extremely muscular to being extremely thin. They may have the characteristic physical traits of mesomorphs such as explained above, but they have an inclination to gain fat typically in the abdominal region of the body. Ecto-mesomorphs can increase the lean muscle tissue in their body through regular resistance training, but unlike mesomorphs they are not generally as strong and explosive in their movements.

Male Endomorphs

Male endomorphs are generally short and stocky and have a lot of fat all over the body. They are typically apple shaped with short necks and with large circumference of waist, ankles and calves. Even if they have good cardiovascular endurance capabilities, male endomorphs find it almost impossible to lose weight. As a result of which they are prone to cardiovascular as well as coronary diseases and even lifestyle diseases such as diabetes.

Female Ectomorph

Female ectomorphs are extremely slim and the measurement is extremely low for hips, shoulders, neck, ankles and calves. Like male-ectomorphs, females have an uncanny tendency to put on whatever little fat they can, in the abdominal region and hips, while the limbs still remain long and slender. Taller women within this category are slightly more athletic in nature but fail to develop any feminine characteristics without the help of intervention through a weight management program. Typically women who fall in this category have high cardiovascular endurance and are good at long duration endurance activities. Among all the categories of women their life span is invariably the longest.

Female Mesomorph

Female mesomorphs are known for their hour-glass shaped physical structure, with wide hips and shoulders but a distinctively narrow waistline. Any weight gain or loss happens proportionally in the upper body – back, shoulders and chest and the lower body – hips and thighs. Women in this category are generally good at certain athletic sports and activities.

Female Meso-Endomorph

Females generally have body fat percentages in the range of 30% which is much higher than that of men. These female meso-endomorphs are much more common than their male counterparts. Females who fall in this category generally have a pear shaped body with wide hips, medium size waist and small shoulders. Such women have a tendency to look unbalances when they go even slightly out of shape. This can easily be corrected through a proper workout program.

Female Endomorphs

Women in this category have larger upper bodies in comparison to the lower half. They have an apple shaped body with large chest and abdomen but narrower hips. These women are prone to putting on weight very easily and that too visceral fat around the organs. This makes the susceptible to cardiovascular diseases and other coronary diseases. It is therefore very important for women who are female endomorphs to ensure that through a weight management system they follow a proper lifestyle which includes exercise, proper nutrition as well as enough rest.

Changes During Puberty

There is a considerable change that the body undergoes during puberty. The difference between the male and the female body starts getting accentuated at this stage. These changes happen for the reproductive reasons. Inherited genetic code plays a big factor in the body shape that starts developing at this stage. The amount of lean muscle mass and the fat distribution pattern along with the skeletal structure all are influenced by the genetic make-up of the individual.

Skeletal Structure

Males on an average are taller and broader in comparison to females. Analysis of body shape though, should be done after taking into consideration the difference in height. Males generally have broad shoulders coupled with wide chest. This happens as a result of testosterone influencing the widening of the rib cage. The reason behind this is that males require more oxygen for fueling the larger muscle mass that is distributed over the body. To facilitate this increased oxygen requirement there needs to be more space for the lungs to pull in more air during respiration, as a result of which expansion of the rib cage happens.

In females at this stage of puberty, widening of hips starts occurring. Estrogen which is the female sex hormone causes the widening of the pelvic girdle specifically for the purposes of childbirth. The larger and rounded pelvic structure allows the fetus head to pass through during child birth. As a result of this widening of the pelvis, the carrying angle of the elbows also increases in comparison to that of men. The sacrum is also wider and shorter and this results in the swaying of hips distinctly visible in the walking style of females. However, these characteristics cannot be stereotyped; both male and female sex hormones are present in each and every individual and the presence of the other se hormone has some effect in determining the body shape and characteristics to a certain extent.

Fat Distribution

Fat distribution plays a significant role in defining the body shape. There is a direct correlation between current fat distribution and sex hormones levels in the body. As can be expected, the skeletal structure does not change after adulthood, but the fat distribution is can be altered by modifying dietary habits and through exercise. As fat distribution changes the shape of the body itself changes visibly.

Contrary to general belief, the right amount of fat in the body is not only acceptable but in fact is necessary for optimal health. In women estrogen causes fat to be deposited in the hips, thighs and buttocks areas. Thus women generally have smaller waists but larger hips, and thus have a lower waist hip ratio in comparison to men. Women also have a much higher body fat percentage as compared to men, this is because the body is prepared for the extra energy requirements that may needed to be met during pregnancy. Post menopause though, the fat distribution in women changes and the fat starts accumulating in the abdominal region itself, as is the case with men. While estrogen promotes storage of fat in the body, testosterone reduces the fat percentage in the body by increasing the metabolic rate.

Females have mammary glands and consequently breasts which start developing after puberty; again due to the effects of estrogen in the body. Testosterone on the contrary helps men build lean muscle tissue in the body which can be enlarged through a proper exercise routine and healthy diet as part of a weight management plan.

Posture & Gait

Body shape also has a defining say in the body posture as well as gait. These play a major role in creating physical attraction. The body shape to a certain extent is representative of the sexual hormones present at that particular point in time as well as that during puberty which points towards fertility. A good body shape apart from being pleasing also implies good health.

Body Types – Effect of Exercise & Diet

As is expected, not each and every one of us is born with the dream physique of a pure mesomorph. Like in sports some people are way more talented than others and find it much easier to excel, in physical exercise too, some people are naturally gifted and find it easier to achieve and maintain a perfectly chiseled body. This is something that is build into the genetic code over which we have no control. An ectomorph might try and eat and workout really very hard but still find it difficult to add lean muscle to the body, whereas endomorphs don't seem to lose any fat which they generally have an excess of, despite following the strictest of weight management plans and the most strenuous of exercise programs.

However, this in no way means that an ectomorph will not gain weight, nor does it mean that an endomorph will not lose fat. It is just that things will be harder than what a pure mesomorph experiences. Further, generally a person is a combination of somatotypes and it is important to first understand the body type before designing a weight management plan which aims for a particular goal or outcome. Once this has been done, adherence to the program is of utmost importance; by following the guidelines over a period of time, one is bound to overcome the genetic disadvantages and achieve the fitness targets that have been set.

Ectomorph

As discussed earlier, these are people who have very little muscle and very little fat in their body. They are also referred to as 'hard gainers' because of their tendency to gain no weight at all despite consuming a heavy diet and exercising. The reason behind this is their extremely high metabolic rate, as a result of which very little storage takes place in the body. The aim is to increase weight by an increase in lean muscle, but even if the ectomorphs eat a heavy diet they put on a little fat around the abdominal region which is most undesirable. By nature too, they do not have the physical endurance and strength that may help them in achieving these goals albeit with extra effort. However, through a proper exercise program this can be altered.

Training for an ectomorph should predominantly be a heavy strength or resistance training program but the macro cycles in the program should be planned in a controlled way since they initially possess very little muscle to perform these workouts and overtraining at this initial stage may lead to injuries jeopardizing the entire program. The focus should be in learning the techniques first and then building up a little endurance and strength both muscular and cardiovascular, before ramping up the intensity. In case this is not done chances of fast burnout may occur and the person leaves the program. A gradual increase in intensity and weight needs to be incorporated as part of the program. This is important from the perspective of program efficiency as well as from the point of view of increased chances of adherence. The following points should be taken into consideration while designing the weight management program for an ectomorph:

1. Exercise duration – The duration of the workout session should not be more than an hour in any case, since the risks of overtraining ectomorphs specially is pretty high. Considering their limited endurance level, fatigue and exhaustion starts setting in earlier than usual during the session and unnecessarily pushing harder will in no way yield results. Contrarily, it only increases the chances of an injury. The goal should be to first increase stamina and then increase the intensity of the workout, perhaps, keeping the duration of workout similar.
2. Exercises – The kind of exercises that are suited for ectomorphs are multi-joint and compound exercises. The aim is to provide an extra stimulus that is responsible for pushing the body to grow further by adding lean muscle tissue. Exercises such as squats, push–ups, pull–ups etc. are extremely useful in creating this stimulus. Not only are these exercises multi-joint but are also compound in nature, involving more than one muscle group. The issue with these exercises is that a person new to strength training will find it difficult initially and may take significant time in learning these exercises. Secondly, a variety of exercises should be used to train each and every muscle group. Since, ectomorphs have very little muscle mass, they will have certain weak areas. For example, it is important to train the entire triceps group through a variety of exercises so that the person may also be able to perform push–ups efficiently. If the triceps are left untrained, then the major muscle group while doing push–ups, chest muscles in this case do not fatigue, but

the smaller supporting muscle, in this case triceps reaches exhaustion. Hence, the exercise no longer remains efficient to train the pectorals. It is therefore crucial to train all muscle groups of the body.

3. Sets – Due to limited lean muscle tissue in the body, the number of sets per exercise should be limited. Rather a variety of exercises should be chosen for the workout session. For each muscle group and at each stage of development of the group, a certain number of sets per exercise is ideal. Once the number of sets crosses this benefits from these sets starts diminishing as well. Generally at the initial stage of the program, not more than 2 to 3 sets per exercise should be performed for each exercise.
4. Repetitions – This refers to the number of times a movement is performed in each set. The goal of any strength training program for an ectomorph is to increase lean muscle mass, this can happen through a process called hypertrophy. For hypertrophy to occur, the number of repetitions per set should be limited between 9 to 12 counts. The number of repetitions has a direct relationship with the resistance or load that is lifted for the exercise. Greater number of repetitions means lower resistance and lesser number of repetitions means that a higher resistance can be chosen. For example, an individual who is performing squats and is able to lift 100 lbs. for 12 repetitions, will be able to lift 150 lbs. in case he or she needs to perform only 6 repetitions whereas the load will go down to 75 lbs. in case the number of repetitions increases to 18. By increasing the repetitions and consequently reducing load, an endurance workout is performed. By decreasing the repetitions and consequently increasing the load a strength workout is performed. The goal for an ectomorph is gain in size or hypertrophy; this can be achieved with around 9 to 12 repetitions per set.
5. Rest between sets – Whenever an exercise is performed energy utilized is in the form of a molecule called ATP or Adenosine Tri Phosphate. This is the only energy molecule in the body that the muscles can utilize to perform work. Metabolism of energy molecules such as carbohydrates, fats and proteins yields ATP which is then utilized. Limited amount of ATP can be stored in the working muscles

therefore as we perform more and more work, ATP needs to be generated. For hypertrophy to take place, rest period between sets should be limited to 45 seconds.

6. Resistance training techniques – Simple linear general training should be performed at the initial stage. This means that in a sequential manner, 2 to 3 sets of each exercise should be performed taking into account the right number of repetitions and the appropriate rest period between the sets. Once a couple of months have passed and the person has learnt the correct techniques, new training protocols such as eccentric training, compound training, tri–sets, rest & pause and super sets can be incorporated as part of the workout. Initially however, things should be kept simple and manageable.
7. Calorie count – An ideal target is a gain of around 1 to 2 lbs. of lean mass per week. To do this, an energy excess of around 750 calories per day needs to be achieved. This energy excess shall be utilized in repair and growth of the muscle tissue that has been utilized during workout. In the absence of any workout, it starts getting stored as fat. Therefore, workout and diet go together in helping an individual achieve his or her fitness goals.
8. Frequency of meals – Ectomorphs have a very high metabolic rate, therefore it is important that the body is fuelled on a regular basis. By performing high intensity exercise, the requirement of the body goes up. In case adequate energy is not provided at the correct time, the body starts utilizing resources from within. This is not desirable since the goal is weight gain and we do not want any loss of weight happening due to inadequate energy being provided to the body. It is therefore important to consume meals every two to three hours so that the body is fuelled at the correct rate to enhance growth.
9. Meal Content – The dietary breakup should be such that all macro nutrients as well as micro nutrients are made available in sufficient quantities. A diet in which the amount of calories derived from carbohydrates is 45%, from proteins is 35% and that from fats is 20% is ideal. A few alterations can be made within this structure to suit individual needs.

10. Pre & Post workout meals – These are extremely important meals of the day and the efficiency of a workout session can double if the right kind of nutrition is made available to the body prior to, during and after the workout. In an ectomorph, the goal is to increase weight by utilizing resources from outside to fuel the requirements of the body. Lesser the dependence on internal sources better it is. Prior to the workout, a combination of complex carbohydrates with some protein source is ideal. This will ensure that the body is gradually provided energy over the duration of the workout. In case an energy deficit is experienced during the workout then during the next workout, pre-workout meal content could be ramped up with an increased amount of carbohydrates. Post workout meal is important since this is when the muscle tissues open up a kind of anabolic or growth window. A combination of simple sugars such as glucose & fructose along with fast acting proteins such as whey seems ideal for the purpose. The insulin spike experienced as a result of glucose entering the blood stream will help in the pushing glycogen into the muscles. Eating at regular intervals after this will provide the right kind of environment for the muscles to grow.
11. Types of food – Apart from the anabolic phase, it is important to consume slow metabolizing foods such as complex carbohydrates and slow acting proteins. This will ensure that storage by conversion into fat is avoided when the body does not require energy at that fast rate. At the same time the energy as well as growth requirements of the body are met.

Along with the right kind of diet and exercise as part of a weight management plan ectomorphs should rest appropriately, since the muscles need time to recover from the strain they have been put under. A combination of these three components of fitness will lead to healthy weight gain in the long duration.

Mesomorphs

Mesomorphs possess the ideal body type. They are generally muscular and athletic with little amount of fat in the body. In case this is not the case, and dude to some reason they have put on fat, still, their natural predisposition is towards losing fat and increasing lean muscle tissue in the body. The genetic build up is such that it is inclined towards a muscular physique with broad shoulders and wider side to side measurement in comparison to front to back measurements. The following points should be taken into consideration while designing a weight management program for a mesomorph:

1. Duration of exercise – Since they possess a physical structure that can endure higher intensities, duration of exercise should generally be an hour but it can go up on certain days which may be kept for heavy endurance training. Even Mesomorphs though can be new to exercise and strength training in particular. It is important to appreciate this fact and go slow in the initial stages of the program. Gradually, the intensity can be increased to higher levels since the body is suited to perform under these circumstances. Understanding the techniques first should be given priority before ramping up the volume & load. It is also important to understand the limits of the body and a number of Mesomorphs commit the mistake of overtraining and putting the body under undue stress.
2. Exercises – Mesomorphs should perform a combination of all exercises. Their workouts in general should cover all aspects of fitness – muscular strength, muscular endurance, cardiovascular endurance and flexibility. There can be specific training goals such as increasing lean mass for bigger physique or improving cardiovascular endurance for long distance running. In these situations workout should be goal specific and should predominantly work towards better performance in that respect, however, other aspect of fitness should also be given due importance for optimal health. A combination of different strength training exercises should be chose. These should include single as well as multi-joint exercises, compound as well as isolated movements. Even for improving cardiovascular endurance a combination of workouts should be chosen such as running, swimming, biking etc. These different exercises though working on cardiovascular endurance utilize different muscle groups and add variety in a manner such that overall fitness of the individual improves.
3. Sets – General training programs should include workout days which concentrate on building up of muscular strength,

increasing muscular endurance as well as sessions for hypertrophy. Such a well rounded macro plan will ensure a good balance. When the goal is hypertrophy the number of sets should increase as increased volume of workout is the requirement. When gaining strength is the goal, number of sets can be moderate to high, while when endurance is the goal, the number of sets per exercise should be moderate.

4. Repetitions – The number of repetitions per set and consequently the resistance or load should also vary depending on the purpose of the workout session. For strength gains the number of repetitions per set is small, in the range of 4 to 6 and load is higher, for hypertrophy number of repetitions is moderate – 9 to 12, and so is the load, and for muscular endurance the number of repetitions is high – 16 to 18 and even more, and load or resistance comes down considerably.
5. Rest between sets – The rest between sets should be kept at around 45 seconds to 1 minute, unless workout is being performed for strength gains. In this case, the rest period can go up to 3 minutes. The reason behind this is that the exercising muscle needs to recover and enough ATP needs to be present in the muscle to perform the exercise for the next set.
6. Training techniques – Unlike ectomorphs and endomorphs, mesomorphs should incorporate a lot of variety in their workouts. Once the technique of training and method or posture for each exercise being performed has been learnt, Mesomorphs should incorporate not only different exercises but also different routines and workout patterns. This ensures that a different stimulus is being provided to the body in each workout and therefore the body improves further over a period of time.
7. Calorie count – Depending on the goal of the individual mesomorph, calorie count can vary. In case a weight gain is desired then energy excess needs to be achieved while if weight loss is desired then energy deficit needs to be created. In general, an excess or a deficit of around 500 calories per day is ideal depending on the goal. This will lead to a weight difference of around 1 to 2 lbs. per week which is a healthy target.

8. Meal frequency – A 6 meal program including pre & post workout meals ensures that the body is provided energy and nutrition when it requires it. It then has no need to store any of this extra energy in the body.
9. Meal content – A balanced nutrition program with the right macro nutrient as well as micro nutrients and anti-oxidants is desired. The percentage of calories from can be in the following ratio: 55–60% from carbohydrates, 15–20% from proteins and 20–25% from fats. A variety of foods should be consumed so that all the necessary vitamins & proteins are made available to the body in the right quantities.
10. Pre & Post workout meals – Pre-workout meal should be such that there is sufficient energy in the body to perform exercises at the intensity that is desired. Post workout meal should be such that it provides ample fuel immediately for growth. As in other cases, the meal content and quantity depends on the goal of the program. Weight loss goals will entail meal patterns such that resources such as stored glycogen and fat are utilized from within the body, while weight gain goals will need meals such that enough energy as well as amino acids from protein break down is made available through a proper diet all throughout the day and specifically immediately after exercise session.

The workout and diet pattern for Mesomorphs is completely dependent on the goal. Since, Mesomorphs in general can have variety of workout objectives, therefore it is important to first understand those goals and then design an appropriate program. Once those goals are achieved Mesomorphs enter maintenance phase which requires a well rounded and balanced workout routine as well as diet program.

Endomorphs

Endomorphs have a large skeletal structure and are predisposed to storing a lot of fat all over the body. They have wide shoulders as well as hips and accumulate lot of fat in the upper arms, thighs as well as abdominal region. Endomorphs have a tendency to gain weight very easily; however, a large portion is undesirable fat and not lean muscle. The program goal for endomorphs is to reduce the body fat percentage drastically. In case of endomorphs who have lost this fat, the aim is them to maintain this at the same time to try and increase lean muscle mass. The following points should be taken into consideration while designing a weight management program for a mesomorph:

1. Duration of exercise – The maximum duration of exercise for endomorphs should be around an hour. There is a tendency to overdo cardiovascular workouts for long durations above the one hour mark. However, this leads to unnecessary loss of lean muscle tissue. There are ways and methods which when applied properly can help in lose fat at the same time prevent the loss of lean muscle tissue to a certain extent. As is the case with other body types the intensity of workouts should increase only gradually once techniques and correct methods to perform exercises have been learnt.
2. Exercises – Endomorphs should perform exercises covering all aspects of fitness but the main attention is towards burning calories through cardiovascular endurance as well as strength training workouts. Aerobic activities such as jogging, swimming, cycling are appropriate cardiovascular workouts. In case the individual is extremely obese, then non–impact activities such as cycling on a recumbent bike are more suitable since the load on the knees is limited. It is also important to understand the concept of heart rate in this regard. Whenever a person exercises the heart rate increases from that at rest. The maximum heart rate of a person is age dependent. Thus, the heart rate can vary between these two levels – resting heart rate and maximum heart rate. The difference between the two is called the heart rate reserve. When a person works out at an intensity corresponding to 40 to 50% of the heart rate reserve then the activity is aerobic in nature. This means that the production of energy happens by metabolism in the presence of oxygen. This is important since fat can be burned only through aerobic methods. As the intensity increases the process becomes anaerobic and fat will no longer be used as the primary source of energy. Thus, exercises should be performed at a moderate intensity to burn fat. This is extremely important to build into

the exercise program. Further, endomorphs should try and burn calories through resistance training workouts as well. Multi-joint compound movements are preferred since they burn more number of calories in comparison to isolated exercises. Also, free weight exercises are preferred in comparison to working out on machines. The reason behind this is that the balance and coordination that is required for free weight exercises require significantly higher neuro-muscular coordination. This means a greater effort and higher number of calories being burnt in the process as well.

3. Sets – The primary training goal of endomorphs is to burn calories and to utilize the stored fat in the body for the purpose. Cardiovascular workouts should be performed for at least 20 to 30 minutes and this can go up as endurance increases and the heart rate continues to remain at a moderate level even at higher intensities and after long durations. For resistance training, the number of sets can be 3 per exercise in such a way that all body parts are worked out over the course of the week. Since the choice of exercises are generally compound in nature that utilize many muscle groups, the chance of leaving out a particular muscle is generally low, but still care should be taken to avoid this.
4. Repetitions – The number of repetitions per set should be kept high since the effort is to burn more calories. This can be from 12 – 15 repetitions per set.
5. Rest between sets – The rest between sets should be kept at around 30 – 45 seconds. In such a situation the heart rate remains elevated even during resistance training workouts and mimics a cardiovascular workout. When the heart rate remains elevated it leads to burning more number of calories throughout the exercise session.
6. Training techniques – Endomorphs can incorporate numerous techniques and workout principles. Ideal ones are those in which exercises are performed back to back with minimal rest between sets. For example, circuit training is a workout principle in which a set of around 10 – 12 exercises of various muscle groups are performed for a specific number of repetitions without rest between exercises. A person moves from one

station to another immediately and does not rest until the entire circuit is completed. Such workouts keep the heart rate at an elevated level, helping the body to burn fat consistently.

7. Calorie count – This particular parameter is most important for endomorphs. The goal is to lose approximately 2 lbs. of fat every week on a continuous basis. This means an energy deficit of around 1,000 calories needs to be created on a daily basis. Thus the intake needs to be carefully measured and monitored.
8. Meal frequency – A high frequency low calorie meal plan is ideal for endomorphs. The body does not require huge amounts of energy at any time during the day. Heavy meals will lead to utilization of a part of the calories ingested and storage as fat of the remaining amount. A weight management diet plan such as 6 meal plan ensures that the body gets only what it requires and when it requires it. There is no storage since there is no excess left after the calories from that meal have been utilized.
9. Meal content – Contrary to numerous myths and popular weight loss diet plans, a balanced nutritious diet is correct for even endomorphs trying to lose weight. The percentage of calories can be in the following ratio – 50–55% from carbohydrates, 20–25% from proteins and 20–25% from fats. A variety of foods should be included in the diet plan so that all the essential micro-nutrients are available for the smooth functioning of the body.
10. Pre & Post workout meals – Pre-workout meal can include a small complex carbohydrate snack that ensures that there is energy in the body to perform the workout. Working out on an empty stomach has numerous issues associated with it and therefore should be avoided. Post workout meal should also consist of complex carbohydrates along with fast acting protein. This means that even after workout when the heart rate remains elevated due to principles like EPOC (excess post-exercise oxygen consumption) the body uses the stored reserves such as body fat for fulfilling this energy requirement.

Endomorphs should be mindful that too much of a cardiovascular workout is not performed and that too at high intensities. The reason for this is that although there will be considerable loss of weight, it will involve loss of lean muscle tissue as well. This situation is not desirable and should be avoided. In most cases, however, there is some amount of muscle loss that happens and once endomorphs have lost the excess fat in the body, the weight management plan should focus on recovering the lost lean muscle tissue in the process.

Irrespective of the type of body that an individual possesses it is possible through a combination of proper diet, exercise and rest to alter the characteristics inherent with the body type. The body type is built into our genetic structure, but that does not mean that the traits associated with the body type are beyond our control. It may require significant amount of effort but it is possible for an endomorph to lose excess fat, and it is possible for an ectomorph to gain lean muscle tissue.

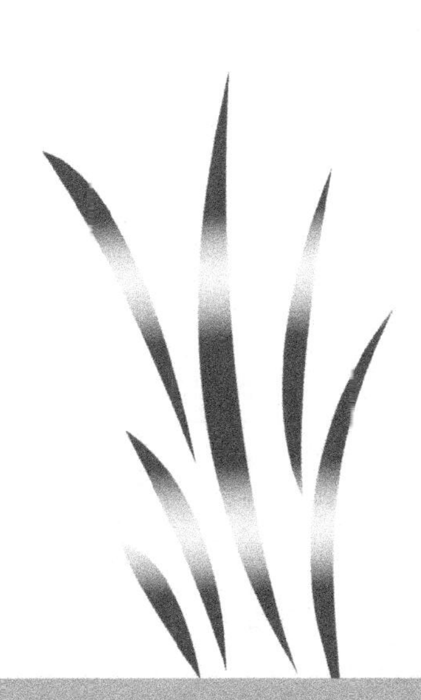

Ideal Body Goals

Ideal Body Goals

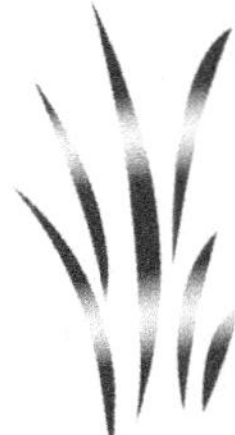

What is Body Weight?

Our Body Weight is the force that the earth exerts on our bodies due to gravitational pull. Everything else remains the same, only the constituent elements in our bodies change causing a change in our body weight. Therefore, let us first understand the composition of the human body.

The human body primarily comprises of water, bones, organs, lean muscle and fat. Within the context of a weight management program, the most important components are lean muscle and fat, since only these can be controlled with proper exercise, diet and nutrition. They can be clubbed together into two basic categories – body fat & fat free weight. Good physical fitness as well as appearance is defined by these two parameters. Low fat percentage in the body and high fat free weight indicate a good body composition.

Body Composition

Body composition analysis refers to the method used to determine the percentage of each of the constituent elements of the body, importantly body fat and lean muscle tissue percentages. There are many methods employed to perform body composition analysis. Traditionally measurement calipers were used to measure the fat in multiple places in the body. This method is cheap and easy to perform but it is not very accurate. Fat itself is of two types – subcutaneous and visceral. Subcutaneous fat is the fat that is present under the skin and is distributed all over the body. Visceral fat is the fat around the organs present for their protection and cushioning. This fat is clearly visible in the abdominal region. The usage of calipers to perform skin fold measurements is based on the principle that fat gets proportionally distributed all over the body. By estimating the total subcutaneous fat, it is possible to determine total body fat percentage.

Hydrostatic weighing is a very accurate method to perform body composition analysis but it is quite cumbersome. Its accuracy is so high that it is sometimes called the gold standard for body composition. It utilizes Archimedes principle to measure body density by immersing the entire body in water. Lean muscle tissue is heavier in comparison to fat, and using the measurement of body density as calculated in hydrostatic weighing it is possible to estimate body fat percentage.

New technologies that are used for body composition analysis include methods such as Bioelectric Impedance Analysis (BIA), Dual Energy X-ray Absorptiometry (DEXA) and Ultrasound. With research & development these methods have now become commercially usable and viable. In common practice, bioelectric impedance analysis and ultrasound are nowadays are commonly used for the purpose. Both BIA and Ultrasound are convenient methods for body composition since they can be performed with high accuracy in a short period of time. Moreover, the equipment used for the purpose is small and portable. BIA uses a small electrical current to flow through the body to calculate electrical resistance. Fat is a bad conductor of electricity. By measuring the magnitude of this resistance or impedance it is possible to estimate fat percentage. Ultrasound uses high frequency sound waves to perform the analysis since the response of fat to ultrasound waves is very different from the response of lean mass in the body. Earlier, body composition analysis was used sparingly for technical studies and research. However, with the requirement posed by the burgeoning fitness and wellness industry, it is now commonly used. There are many advantages of performing body composition analysis on a regular basis.

- It helps in determining the health status of the member by calculating the fat mass and lean muscle mass. Greater the lean muscle mass healthier is the individual. Lesser the fat mass healthier is the individual.
- It helps the exercise programmer in designing the exercise card and the nutrition counselor to prepare a diet plan on the basis of the analysis. The target of fitness programs is to increase lean muscle tissue and decrease fat percentage.
- Body composition analysis done on a regular basis helps in determining the progress of a weight management program. Changes can be introduced in the program after analyzing the effects of the previous exercise program and diet plan on the body composition.

A typical body composition analysis provides a lot of information and measures numerous different parameters. The parameters that are most important to analyze include the following:

1. **Weight** – It is the total body weight in kilograms or pounds.
2. **Skeletal Muscle Mass (SMM)** – It is the total weight of lean muscle tissue in the body expressed in kilograms or pounds.
3. **Body Fat Mass** – It is the total fat mass measured in kilograms or pounds. It includes both the subcutaneous fat and visceral fat
4. **Fat Free Mass** – It is the total weight of the non-fat part of the body. (Fat Free Mass = Weight – Body Fat Mass). It is measured in kilograms or pounds.
5. **Body Mass Index (BMI)** – It is a value which is used to classify whether the person is obese, overweight, underweight or normal. It is commonly used as the parameter when body composition analyzers are not available. It is like a thumb rule and tells us with a simple arithmetic calculation, as to which category a person belongs to. *BMI = (Weight in Kilograms)/(Height in meters)*^{2}. BMI works well in most cases however, it only takes into consideration body weight (height of a person is assumed to be constant after adulthood). BMI calculations will classify a body builder as obese, since the body weight will be higher despite most of it being lean muscle and not fat. In such cases where distinction between fat and lean mass is important, BMI does not provide the correct results. It is therefore imperative to measure body fat and lean muscle percentages separately.
6. **Percentage Body Fat** – It is the body fat mass expressed as a percentage of body weight. Percentage Body Fat = {(Body Fat Mass)/(Weight)}*100. This is the most useful as well as important parameter that is used while designing a weight management program. In general, males have a body fat percentage in the range of 10 to 20%. In females due to the sex hormone estrogen, body fat percentage is higher in the range of 20 to 30%.
7. **Resting Metabolic Rate (RMR)** – It is the calories that the body burns in a complete state of rest in a day for essential processes such as respiration and digestion. Greater the

lean muscle mass in the body greater will be the BMR, and hence the body will be able to burn more number of calories throughout the day.

The Body Composition analysis also gives a segmental analysis of the fat mass and lean muscle tissue in the body. It calculates the mass of fat and lean muscle in the left arm, right arm, left leg, right leg and trunk. This information may be utilized in case there are fitness goals that are specifically related to increase in lean muscle and consequently weight gain. Segmental analysis may not be too useful for weight loss, since the aim is to reduce the body fat percentage. As fat is present throughout the body, the proportion in which fat loss happens is commensurate to this distribution. Contrary to popular myth, spot reduction of fat cannot take place since fat is an energy substrate that will reduce when it is used for metabolism for production of energy that the body requires.

Overweight & Obesity

The weight of an individual should be within a particular prescribed range. This range typically measured as percentage of body fat depends on parameters such as age, sex, height etc. When the fat percentage in the body is above the prescribed range, the person is said to be overweight. A certain basic amount of fat is required in the body for essential functions such as protection of organs and temperature regulation, but when the percentage goes beyond the range then it starts having detrimental effects on the body. When the percentage of body fat goes even higher, the individual is said to be obese. Obesity is one of the most common lifestyle diseases plaguing the world population. Over a billion people in the world are either overweight or are obese and more than 60% of the adult population in Unite States of America falls under this classification. Despite the level of awareness going up on a continuous basis, the prevalence of obesity has been on the rise over the past many years. Obesity puts the individual at high risk to numerous health issues such as coronary and cardiovascular disease, diabetes and other chronic ailments thereby drastically reducing life expectancy. In the ages gone by being overweight or obese was considered to be a sign of wealth over the years there has been a cultural swing with people now understanding the issues associated with being overweight and obese. It is also manifested in the fact that being overweight or obese is not considered physically appealing any more, and being slim and looking fit is far more preferable.

A common quick thumb rule that can be used for determining whether a person is overweight or obese is Body Mass Index. In case the BMI of a person is more than 25 the person is classified as being overweight while in case it goes above 30, the person is said to be obese. There are various degrees or levels of obesity – level 1 to 3 and specifies the extent of obesity in the individual with a BMI which is greater than 40 is classified as morbid obesity. The exact number range is defined by World Health Organization but other health bodies have made certain modification to suit specific populations since ethnicity also has a role to play in the way obesity is classified as well as the way in which the problem is approached. For example, the negative impact of excess fat percentage is greater at lower levels of BMI in case of Asian population in comparison to Caucasians. As a result of this, in Asian countries, the range for classification as obese starts at 25 itself. As mentioned earlier as well, it is important to understand that BMI is only an indicator and may not be accurate in specific cases such as when body weight is high but lean muscle tissue is greater and fat percentage is pretty low. In terms of body fat percentage, the normal range is 20 to 30% for females and 10 to 20% among males. A person is said to be obese when the fat percentage in the body goes above the upper limit of the range. Body fat percentage is a more accurate indicator, but BMI is in common practice because of ease of measurement and calculation.

Spread of Obesity

Overweight and Obesity expose the individual to numerous risk factors, and is now globally considered fifth in the list of risks leading to death. According to WHO around 3 million people die each year through indirect effects of being overweight or obese. There are more than 1.6 billion adults who are overweight with around 10% of the global population classified in the obese category. The distribution in terms of sex is more or less even with the around 40% of the obese category being males 60% of the category as females. The problem exists even with children; for children under the age of five, close to 45 million lie in the overweight category with more than 80% of these children living in under–developed and developing countries of the world.

In the United States of America, according to NHANES, 33% of adults (over the age of 20 years) are overweight, 35.7% are classified as being obese and 6.3% in the morbid obesity category. Since the late 1980s there has been a steady increase in percentage of the adult population in the obese category, rising from around 23% in 1988 to more than 36% as on date. In the last decade, this percentage of obese women has remained more or less the same, while it has steadily increased in a linear fashion for men. During the period from 1980 to 2010, while the percentage of obese people more than doubled, the percentage of people in the overweight category more or less remained the same.

There is no significant variation in the change in percentage of obese males within various ethnic groups. For non-Hispanic white men, the percentage jumped from 20.3% in 1988 to 36.2% in 2012; for non-Hispanic black men, it jumped from 21.1% in 1988 to 38.8% in 2012; for Mexican- American men, it jumped from 23.9% in 1988 to 36.6% in 2012. As can be observed there is no significant variation in case of males. However, in case of females a stark difference is seen for non-Hispanic black women. For non-Hispanic white women, the percentage jumped from 22.9% in 1988 to 32.2% in 2012; for non-Hispanic black women, it jumped from 38.4% in 1988 to 58.5% in 2012; for Mexican- American women, it jumped from 35.4% in 1988 to 44.9% in 2012.

Obesity in children also called childhood obesity is also posing a significant global problem. Steadily but surely the percentage of children who are overweight and obese has gone up attaining significant proportions. In the United States of America, according to a NHANES study conducted in 2009-10, 16.9% of all children in the age group 2 to 19 were obese. If we look at the break-up, for children in the age group 2 to 5 years, the percentage of obese children increased from 5% in 1980 to 12.1% in 2010; for children in the age category 6 to 11, this percentage increased from 6.5% in 1980 to 18.0% in 2010; for children in the age category 12 to 19 this percentage increased from 5% in 1980 to 18.4% in 2010. If we study the last decade in isolation, for boys there was a significant increase in percentage who were obese, but it remained more or less the same in case of girls.

The number of older adults, defined as people over the age of 65 in the United States of America is expected to double by the year 2050. In terms of numbers, the expected increase is from around 43 million to about 88 million. This increase is due to a combination of an increase in population and the availability of better and more advanced medical facilities and services thereby improving life expectancy. Around 35% of people in the older adult category were obese in 2010. This corresponded to 8 million in the age group 65 to 74, roughly 40.8% of this category and about 5 million in the age group 75 and above, which is approximately 27.8% of the category. Over the last decade the percentage of obese males in the 65 to 74 age category has gone up from 31.6% in 2000 to 41.5% in 2010. For the above 75 age group category the increase was from 17.7% in 2000 to 26.5% in 2010. During this duration, the change in percentages among females was not significant.

In terms of ethnic background, the observation was contrary to the above case. The difference in males of this age group was not so significant. However, among women – in the age group 65 to 74 years, 53.9% of non-Hispanic black women were obese, 38.9 % of non-Hispanic white women and 46.6% for Hispanic women. In the age group 75 years and above, 49.4% of non-Hispanic black women were obese, 27.5% of non-Hispanic white women and 30.2% for Hispanic women. As can be seen ethnic differences translated into genetic as well as social & cultural reasons has significant impact on obesity levels.

Effects of Obesity On Health

Obesity is called the silent killer. It may not directly lead to death in the manner other disease do, but it indirectly leads to numerous chronic ailments and issues that reduce life expectancy. It is one of the most preventable reasons for death. It has been established in numerous studies that people with low BMI levels are at a lower mortality risk in comparison to those with higher BMI. In the United States alone, about half a million deaths occur every year due to obesity related issues. On an average life expectancy goes down by around two years in case a person is overweight and up to ten years in case of morbid obesity.

Obesity is known to increase the risk of numerous physical, mental and emotional problems. In some cases obesity is directly responsible for manifestation of these chronic ailments, while in others, the correlation is strong because of common causes such as inadequate physical activity, poor diet & nutritional habits and overall sedentary lifestyle. In general, the diseases correlated with obesity can be classified into two basic categories – diseases that occur due to an increase in fat mass and disease that occur due to increase in the number of fat cells in the body. The first category includes osteoarthritis, social isolation and sleep apnea, while the second category includes diseases such as cardiovascular diseases, cancer and diabetes. The most common ailments that are associated with or are correlated with obesity areas following:

1. Type 2 Diabetes - More than 80% of type 2 diabetes patients are overweight or obese. This correlation occurs in men and women alike. This form of diabetes arises when the pancreas stops producing adequate amount of insulin or the cells in the body are not able to utilize the insulin that has been secreted by the pancreas. Whenever there is an increase in sugar level in the blood, pancreas secretes the hormone insulin to help in its metabolism. Obesity severely limits the capacity of insulin to control blood sugar level. As a result of this the body starts to secrete more and more insulin to keep up with the increased blood sugar level, but in the end it is not able to keep the level in range any longer.
2. Cardiovascular & Neurological diseases – Obese people are at high risk to cardiovascular and heart diseases such as myocardial ischemia or heart attack, angina pectoris, congestive heart failure and arrhythmia. This is because they are prone to increased LDL Cholesterol and triglyceride levels in the blood along with their tendency to develop hypertension or high blood pressure. These are the main ingredients that lead to coronary and cardiovascular diseases. Heart attacks are caused by blockages created in the artery that provides oxygen to the myocardial muscles. These symptoms also lead to stroke which occurs when inadequate amount of oxygen reaches the brain. Excess visceral fat or the fat in the abdominal region leads to blood vessels getting inflamed which further raise the risk of these diseases. In the United States coronary artery disease and stroke are the leading causes of death.

3. Hypertension – The blood flowing in the arteries exerts pressure on the arterial wall. This pressure is measured as the blood pressure. Obesity has a direct correlation with blood pressure levels. Individuals already having high blood pressure can see dramatic decrease in the blood pressure levels by decreasing body weight.
4. Metabolic syndrome – It is a group of disorders that which when occur together increase drastically the risk of developing cardiovascular diseases as well as diabetes. These factors include android or central obesity, increased blood pressure, increased blood sugar level, reduced HDL Cholesterol level and increased triglyceride level in the blood. Metabolic syndrome is one of the biggest obesity related issues in the country. Almost 22% of the adult population suffers from metabolic syndrome, in terms of numbers it translates to more than 50 million people.
5. Polycystic Ovary syndrome – It is one of the most common issues faced by women of reproductive age. A majority of these women are overweight and obese. In this syndrome underdeveloped follicles get accumulated in the ovaries leading to menstrual cycles being irregular, above normal hair growth and ovarian cysts. It leads to insulin resistance putting women with this problem at a risk of developing diabetes at a later stage. Even in adolescent girls, high insulin level in the blood, resistance to insulin and obesity are all related to PCOS.
6. Dyslipidemia - It is the condition in which the lipid profile of the blood becomes adverse – HDL cholesterol or the good cholesterol goes down, while triglyceride and LDL cholesterol or the bad cholesterol increases. This is often a result of increase in weight and results in coronary artery disease. Losing weight has a direct correlation with improvement in lipid profile.
7. Gastrointestinal problems
    a. Cholelithiasis – Commonly called gallstones happens when high cholesterol content leads to hardening of bile. These hard, rock like pieces cause severe back and abdominal back pain. In some cases even surgical intervention may be required to remove the gall stones.

b. GERD or Gastroesophageal reflex disease – It is a disease in which the muscles at the bottom of the esophagus allows the stomach contents along with other digestive juices to enter the esophagus

c. Fatty Liver Disease – In this disease fat builds up in the liver leading to inflammation and damages the liver severely by forming fibrous tissues. In some severe cases it can lead to irreversible liver damage as well as liver cirrhosis.

d. Colon cancer – This kind of cancer leads to cancerous kind of growth in the colon, appendix and the rectum.

e. Hernia – The contents of certain body cavities bulge out from their normal areas in hernia. The content includes fatty tissue enclosed in very thin layers or membranes

8. Genitourinary problems

   a. Erectile dysfunction is the inability to maintain an erection of the penis in order for sexual intercourse

   b. Renal failure – This is chronic in nature when the kidneys fail to perform their main function – excreting waste material from the body.

   c. Incontinence – Reduced bladder control leading to slight amount of leakage of urine and also to uncontrolled wetting in severe cases

   d. Hypogonadism – The hormonal production of the sex organs of the body become greatly diminished or my stop completely

   e. Other such problems include uterine and breast cancer, which refers to cancerous growth in the uterus and breast

9. Respiratory problems

   a. Sleep Apnea – The person suffering from this disorder experiences repeated pauses in breathing during sleep. This may occur multiple times and may last for many breaths.

   b. Hypoventilation syndrome – The person facing this disorder does not get enough oxygen during sleep.

This results in high carbon dioxide levels in the blood and consequently low oxygen levels.

c. Dyspnea – This refers to the gamut of disorders that result in shortness of breath manifested by extreme difficulty in breathing

10. Musculoskeletal problems

    a. Osteoarthritis – It is a disease that affects the joints of the body, commonly the knees, lower back and hips. It occurs due to wearing away of the protective cartilage around the joints. Due to obesity there is extra load on these weight carrying joints and the extent of the disorder aggravates further.

11. Psychological problems

    a. Depression – An obese individual may undergo severe bouts of depression wherein there may be a perennial feeling of sadness and hopelessness.

    b. Diminished self confidence – People who are obese and due to various reasons have not been successful in reducing their weight may have extremely low self esteem and low self confidence and this feeling gets stronger as once fails repeatedly in the effort.

Causes of Obesity

Obesity in general is caused by an excess intake of energy through a combination of improper diet and inadequate physical activity. There may however, also be contributing elements such as genetics, medical conditions and disorders. However, this lack of energy balance is the underlying reason behind weight gain. This happens when energy input in the form of food provides more energy than that is expended as energy output by the body. Energy output is a combination of a number of factors.

1. Resting Metabolic Rate (RMR) – It is the total number of calories that the body is able to burn at a state of rest in a day for essential activities of daily life such as respiration, digestion etc.
2. Cost of Activity (COA) – It refers to the total calories that an individual may burn in a day owing to his or her

activities of daily life. These include energy burnt during work. Therefore, a person working an office may burn only 300 calories in an entire working day, while a person who is a supervisor of a real estate firm on the field, will burn at least 600 calories is a day.

3. Cost of Exercise (COE) – It is the calories that a person burns while participating in physical activities such as walking, jogging, swimming and exercising in a gym. This will include energy burnt doing cardiovascular endurance workouts as well resistance training workouts.
4. Thermic Effect of Food (TEF) – Our body requires some energy for breaking down food to release energy. However, some foods such as glucose are absorbed easily while complex compounds like protein require energy to break down and be utilized. Therefore, what is consumed plays an essential role in calculation of Thermic effect of Food.
5. Other factors – Certain other parameters play a very minor role. For example, adaptive thermogenesis is the regulation of heat production in the body as a result of changes in the external environment, this leads to greater inefficiency in metabolism. Shivering in the cold is a distinct example of adaptive thermogenesis. For all practical purposes the magnitude of this is very small and we do not take it into consideration for calculation of energy output.

The net sum of all these parameters is energy output. The total energy released as a result of metabolism of food that has been ingested is energy input. Our diet is a combination of energy compounds that release energy during metabolism; it also should include micronutrients such as vitamins & minerals that are required in small quantities to act as catalysts in various biochemical reactions in the body; finally water and fiber also play an important role in our body and should be consumed in adequate quantities. However, for calculation of energy input we consider the energy released from the breakdown of energy compounds that are consumed as part of the weight management diet plan.

1. 1 gram of carbohydrate releases 4 calories of energy
2. 1 gram of protein releases 4 calories of energy

3. 1 gram of fat releases 9 calories of energy
4. 1 gram of alcohol releases 7 calories of energy

A simple arithmetic exercise will tell us the net calorie intake during the day – this is essentially the energy input component. When energy output is less than energy input then there is energy excess in the body. As can be expected, the body stores this excess energy in the body for utilization during times when there may not be enough energy input to the body. This is the primary cause of weight gain and there are numerous reasons as to why this energy input is greater than energy output that creates this imbalance that leads to weight gain.

Diet

When energy input is more than energy output, weight gain results. Energy input is nothing but the food we ingest. When we eat more food that releases more energy than what we require, it gets stored in the body. Some part of this excess is stored in the form of glycogen in the liver and muscles, but after this it is predominantly stored as fat. This results in a person being overweight initially which then translates in to obesity in case the situation is not controlled. Over the last two decades it has been seen that the increase in percentage of obese people in the adult population of United States has been matched by an increase in the average calorie intake per capita per day. The increase in women was around 350 calories per day while that for men was 170 calories per day. All this extra energy being consumed comes primarily from simple carbohydrates from junk and convenience foods. Consumption of refined high fat food along with sweetened beverages is the primary contributors of this increase in calories per day. The dependence of the average population on these easily available convenience products has increased considerably.

Sedentary Lifestyle

Over the years there has been a big shift away from work that is physically demanding. With the mechanization of almost all kinds of physical work, working hours of most individuals involve hardly any physical labor. For example, in agricultural practices, the demand for physical labor which was quite significant has drastically come down with advent of machines that complete all jobs from harvesting to threshing by the press of a few buttons. In addition the propensity towards leisure activities that provide no physical exercise whatsoever, such playing computer games. Children as well as adults no longer indulge in recreation activities, and even if they do, physically challenging activities are not preferred. In children this lack of adequate physical activity is leading to an increased incidence in the cases of childhood obesity. It is one of the rapidly growing problems of American society and needs to be addressed soon, since childhood obesity translates into various ailments and disorders at a very early stage in life. Consequently, both life expectancy and quality of life diminish rapidly. Sedentary lifestyle has in this manner reduced the energy output component of the equation leading to the imbalance that causes obesity.

Genetics

The link between genetics and obesity has been well researched and documented. Studies have shown that genes have a significant contribution towards weight gain, in both direct as well as indirect ways. Genes have a direct effect on hormonal secretion, insulin resistance, metabolic rate etc. These parameters have an important contribution in the energy balance equation. Indirectly, genes have a significant influence on habits and lifestyle pattern which leads to choices being made that eventually effect the energy balance equation. Studies that have been done on inheritance patterns have concluded that the offspring of two obese people will in more than 75% of the cases be obese. In stark contrast this figure is only 10% in case both the parents have normal weight. Genes also play a significant role in determining where in the body, the extra fat will be stored. A study of body shapes revealed that there is significant correlation between body type and shape of parent and offspring.

Medical Conditions

Numerous medical conditions and disorders lead to the individual being overweight and obese. Hypothyroidism or low activity level of thyroid gland results in low levels of secretion of the thyroid hormone which is essentially a growth hormone. This has a significant influence on the metabolic rate of the body. When insufficient hormone is released it leads to low metabolic rate and consequently the person feels extremely weak. Even after a complete night's sleep the person gets up in a partial state of fatigue. Lethargy and sluggishness is experienced throughout the day. All these factors especially low metabolic rate contribute in weight gain. Polycystic ovarian syndrome or PCOS is a common occurrence in women of reproductive age. Women with PCOS face problems of excessive hair growth and other reproductive issues along with the problem of weight gain. Another example is Cushing's syndrome in which excess cortisone hormone is secreted by the adrenal glands of the body. People with this syndrome gain weight rapidly and tend to store a lot of fat in the upper body typically abdomen, face and neck while still having thin limbs. This syndrome may develop in case high doses of medication such as prednisone are consumed over a period of time. The risk of obesity is seen to be higher in patients with one or the other psychiatric disorders. Numerous medications are also known to cause significant gains in weight. These include antidepressants, antipsychotics, hormones such as insulin, anticonvulsants and some hormonal contraception.

Social Causes

Societal changes over the last few generations have in general been responsible directly and indirectly in increasing the spread of obesity. Culturally being obese and overweight was seen as a sign of great wealth. With the understanding of the correlation of obesity with numerous ailments and diseases a significant cultural shift has taken place against obesity. A shift in attraction has taken place from a well rounded body to one which is slim and physically fit. Such a body is considered appealing and desired by most people, this is due to a change in outlook of the society at large.

Inequities presented by social classes have been posited as an important factor in the increase in obesity in both developed and developing nations of the world. In developed societies, people with wealth are in a position to afford nutritious food and are at leisure to choose activities that involve physical fitness. On the other hand in developing as well as under-developed countries of the world, lack of money forcing purchase of high energy foods, lack of leisure time because of survival pressure and general attitude towards body shape, mass and appearance has lead to a rapid increase in obesity levels.

Other Reasons

A study conducted a few years back listed a set of various reasons that cause obesity other than the commonly known and accepted ones. These include emotional factors such as stress, anxiety and boredom which may lead to an individual eating without being hungry; late pregnancies that may lead to childhood obesity in the child; women finding it difficult to lose weight that has been gained to support the baby during pregnancy; environmental pollutants such as endocrine disruptors that hamper lipid metabolism in the body; with the advancement of age, there is significant loss of lean muscle mass leading to a reduction in metabolism leading to weight gain; insufficient sleep results in an imbalance in the secretion of hormones *ghrelin* (lack of sleep leads to an increase in this hormone which increases hunger), *leptin* (inadequate sleep leads to a decrease in this hormone which gives a feeling of fullness) and insulin (regulates blood sugar level) that leads to weight gain; other genetic factors that are passed on through generations. There may not be conclusive evidence that these factors are responsible for obesity, but empirical studies provide a reasonably high correlation factor between the cause and the effect.

Weight Management

Weight management refers to the group of activities that are performed to gain weight, lose weight or even maintain it at the same level. As described in the previous sections, the goal of weight management programs is to increase lean muscle tissue in case weight gain is desired and to lose fat in case weight loss in the goal. Any weight management program that causes weight alterations to happen in any other manner compromises health to a certain degree. For example, crash dieting is a common practice for losing weight rapidly. This technique involves going on very low calorie diets making the body burn energy reserves from within rather than depending on resources from food that is eaten. Such a weight management plan will definitely lead to weight loss, but this loss of weight will not be healthy. There will be some loss of fat from the body but the body will lose considerable amount of lean muscle tissue as well. Also, the rate at which weight loss happens should be taken into consideration. A benchmark for healthy weight loss or weight gain is 1 to 2 pounds per week. This will ensure that the body does not have to undergo sudden drastic changes. The effect of weight loss is not just manifested in physical appearances but there are quite a few changes that occur within the body, such as changes in metabolic rate which is directly controlled by the hormonal system. These sudden changes therefore should be avoided for healthy weight loss. Another example is the usage of equipment such as sauna belts. These fancy gadgets became very popular in a very short period of time. The sales campaigns projected the product as a messiah in the fight for weight loss. Since it promised immediate weight loss and showed results to back up the claim, people started using it on a regular basis. The usage of these belts not only leads to weight loss but also to inch loss in specific areas of the body where it is used, such as thighs and abdomen. However, the story is quite different when we take a closer look at it. These belts work by increasing temperature and thereby causing perspiration. This loss of water from the body is what is manifested as weight loss and specifically inch loss. Water is one of the most important constituent elements in the body and makes up a high percentage of our blood. It is responsible for transport of oxygen, nutrients, hormones etc. to and from different parts of the body. The effects of dehydration have been well documented and even experienced by each and every one of us. The call of thirst is a sign that the body is on its way to dehydration. Severe dehydration can also lead to death. In such a perspective, it is apparent that the weight loss caused by dehydration can in no way be deemed healthy at all. Thus, although such products give desired results but the ways in which these results are achieved jeopardize health and safety.

A weight management program can never be a product, in the basic sense that it has to be different for each and every individual. The body composition as well as genetic makeup of each and every one of us is different and so each and every program to alter it will also be different. A program can only be effective as well as healthy when it is customized or tailored for the individual to meet the body's specific requirements. In fact, if all measurable parameters such as body composition remain the same, still the response of one individual versus another to exactly the same program will be different. It is therefore imperative that a weight management program be designed, implemented and manipulated taking into consideration the unique requirements and responses of the individual to it.

Components of Weight Management Program

A healthy weight management program aims to achieve and subsequently maintain optimal body weight. This is done by making healthy lifestyle choices such as participating in a regular physical fitness program, eating a nutritious and balanced diet and taking adequate amount of rest during the day. Each of these components is important in the success of the weight management program. In some cases, a person may not be in a position to make the necessary lifestyle changes that are essential for weigh management. For such cases, medication and surgical treatments are available for the treatment of the problem.

Goal Setting

It is extremely important that the first step in any weight management program be taken with utmost care. Goals should be realistic in nature and at the same time it should be ensured that goals do not compromise health in any manner. The following points should be taken into consideration while setting goals.

1. Adults seeking to lose weight should aim to keep the rate of loss of body weight to 1 to 2 pounds per week. Firstly, this weight loss should happen through loss of body fat and not through loss of lean muscle tissue or water. In case a person loses more weight than this, there are good chances that the loss is happening through the unwanted routes. In any case, regular body composition would provide the true nature of the results and adequate intervention in the weight management program can be introduced after analyzing the results. Secondly, gradual weight loss is imperative since a number of hormonal changes follow weight loss and it is important to give the body time to adjust accordingly.

2. Along with 1 to 2 pound per week thumb rule adults should set goals in the range of loss of 5 to 10% of body weight over a 6 month period. This is a healthy rate and lowers the risk of cardiovascular and coronary artery diseases considerably. After a stabilization period following loss of 10% of body weight, in case the individual is still overweight, further weight loss can be planned.
3. In case of children, the focus should be on getting the child involved in physical activities of one form or the other. The child should also be encouraged to eat healthier. Forcing weight loss goals and making the program objective is not suggested in case of children. In case there is an underlying medical condition that may be the reason for the child being overweight or obese, the involvement of a specialist in the field is often beneficial.

Diet Regulation

By regulating the energy intake as part of the weight management program, it is possible to create the energy deficit that is required for weight loss to take place. For burning 1 pound of fat, a deficit of 3,500 calories needs to be created. This means that the difference between energy input and energy output should be 3,500 calories. This will roughly translate into 500 calories per day. Therefore, if the total energy output is 2,000 calories, then the input should be planned in such a manner that the intake does not exceed 1,500 calories. Other important points that should be taken into consideration while preparing a weight management meal plan include:

1. In general, for most women a diet plan providing 1,200 calorie and for most men a plan providing 1,500 calories is sufficient to cause healthy weight loss. In case the individual feels very hungry while following such a weight management plan, then an increase of about 200 calories can be done and then gradually this can be brought back down to calculated levels.
2. Very low calorie diets and crash dieting should not be indulged in. Apart from the loss of lean muscle tissue in the body, it may even lead to an increase of fat storage in the body. Since fat is an energy dense molecule, the body

will go into starvation mode and try and conserve fat at the expense of lean muscle which is difficult to maintain. Further, these low calorie diets may cause other health issues due to lack of proper nutrition being provided for the body.

3. For children and teenagers, the calorie content of food should not be too low. The emphasis should be on eating healthy. In case calorie content of the meals goes below a certain level, it starts hampering the growth of the body which is absolutely undesirable.

4. A balanced and nutritious diet should never be compromised upon. All the macro and micro nutrients have a specific role to play in the proper functioning of the body and the absence or deficiency of even one of these nutrients may lead to medical disorders and consequently be detrimental to overall health. In general, the nutrients can be segregated into 3 categories. The first category includes energy compounds that provide energy to the body when they undergo metabolism – carbohydrates, proteins and fats. The second category includes micro nutrients that are required in small quantities to act as catalysts in various biochemical reactions of the body – vitamins & minerals. The third category includes water & fiber which apart from helping in the digestion of food play other important roles in the body as well. The following points need to be considered while preparing a weight loss meal plan for an individual looking to lose weight.

    a. The diet should be balanced in such a manner that all the nutrients are made available in adequate quantities for the optimal functioning of the body. For micro nutrients, a reference index such as Daily Value (DV) or Recommended Dietary Allowance (RDA) can be used for calculating the amounts in which all these nutrients should be consumed.

    b. The variation in the quantities of energy compounds – carbohydrates, fats and proteins depends on the fitness goals of the individual. Specifically, the quantities are dependent upon whether the person wants to gain or lose weight and also on the rate at which this is desired. In general, 50 to 60% of the energy requirement of the body should be met from carbohydrates, around 20 to 30% from fats and 15 to 20% from proteins. Apart from providing energy, these macro nutrients have other important roles to play in the body and therefore presence in these adequate quantities is deemed imperative.

c. Water should be consumed in adequate quantities; 2 to 3 liters per day is a good amount. This may however vary depending on the environment and parameters such as altitude, humidity and temperature. Fiber is important for digestion and proper amounts should be ingested. 25 to 35 grams of fiber per day is meets the daily requirements of the body.

d. The body requires energy at a particular rate. In case more energy is available at a particular point in time than what it can utilize it starts storing this energy in the form of fat. This is the primary reason why heavy meals should be avoided. Instead, an individual looking to lose weight should go in for low calorie high frequency meals. Following a 6 meal plan ensures that the body is provided enough nourishment, at the same time it does not convert and store the extra energy as fat.

e. Foods that need to be avoided include simple carbohydrates such as sucrose or sugar and glucose which release energy instantly and in case the body does not require the energy it converts the excess and stores it in the form of body fat. Foods rich in trans-fat, saturated fat and cholesterol should be avoided since taking them in large quantities lead to cardiovascular and coronary artery diseases. These include red meat, meat of organs such as liver, dairy products which are high in fat content such as cream and butter, coconut and palm oil, food such as fries cooked in partially hydrogenated oils, egg yolk, and shrimp.

f. Food that can be used as substitutes include canola oil, olive oil, low fat dairy products, lean protein sources such as fish and chicken breast, whole grain foods and plenty of vegetables & fruits.

Physical Activity

Physical activity will increase the energy output that is achieved on a daily basis and help create an energy deficit. This energy deficit will ultimately help in losing weight. Apart from this primary benefit other benefits of regular physical activity include the following:

1. Regular cardiovascular endurance workout helps in improving the efficiency of the cardiovascular system which is responsible for oxygen delivery and utilization in working muscles of the body. It also improves the functioning of the heart leading to chronic adaptations such as lowering of resting heart rate. The functioning of lungs is also positively affected by regular cardiovascular activity.
2. It helps in reduction of risks of cardiovascular disease, coronary artery disease, diabetes, hypertension and cancers
3. Resistance training helps in increasing the lean muscle tissue in the body and also helps in strengthening the joints. Since form of bones follow functionality, resistance training imparts enough stimulus on the bones to strengthen them and also reduce the rate at which loss of bone mineral density occurs.
4. Flexibility training helps improve the range of motion about the joints and prevents injuries that seem to occur fairly commonly in individuals with poor flexibility.
5. Regular exercise helps in improving quality of sleep and also helps the mind to cope with stressful conditions in a better manner.

The major components of an exercise program include muscular strength, muscular endurance, cardiovascular endurance and flexibility. Whatever the goals of the exercise program may be, it is imperative to include all these components of exercise in a program for optimal fitness. In general, a balanced workout program for weight loss should include 30 to 40 minutes of cardiovascular aerobic activity for at least 3 times a week such that heart rate is at moderate levels, resistance training for 2 to 3 times in a week for all major muscle groups such that each group is covered at least once during the week and flexibility training in the form of static stretching for at least 2 to 3 times in a week. The program should be such that the intensity is not increased beyond the comfort level of the participant until and unless all the techniques of exercise are properly learnt. The intensity of the program should increase gradually and can be achieved through progressive overloading leading to improved results. Children should participate in different activities for at least an hour on a daily basis. This should predominantly be aerobic in nature and can include a variety of exercises. However, resistance training with heavy weights should be avoided completely, since this may hamper the growth process of the bones.

Behavioral Changes

To achieve success in weight management programs it is important to introduce behavioral changes to make it conducive for the participant to adhere to the program. The following steps can help immensely in this process:

1. A change in surroundings plays a big role in improving adherence to the program. Simple steps include avoiding eating in front of the television; this leads to overeating since the person is not generally concentrating on what is being eaten. A change of clothes can be carried to work in case exercise is possible close to the workplace, since coming back home after work and then going out to exercise again may be difficult to do. Instead of unhealthy snacks being readily available all around the house, it is better to substitute these with health snacks and salads, so that even if hunger pangs are experienced and food is eaten against the plan, only healthy options are available for consumption.
2. It is important to keep a log while following a weight management plan both for diet as well as for exercise. This helps in understanding what works and what does not work well within the program. Also, it helps in analyzing the program results objectively.
3. It is important to consult experts in the field of nutrition as well as exercise physiology, especially in case there is

an underlying medical condition which may have resulted in weight gain. Also, in case of any contraindications, exercise should be avoided and it should in no case be performed without the consent of a health specialist.

4. A reward system should be part of any weight management program, since it helps in creating the right environment and motivates the person to adhere to the program.

Medication

In certain cases when lifestyle changes may not be possible to incorporate, such as when due to an underlying medical condition, a person may not be able to perform physical exercise or when a person is morbidly obese and cannot even walk properly, medication for weight loss may be prescribed. A few FDA approved drugs that are used for weight loss include the following:

1. Orlistat can be used to lose weight in the range of around 5 to 10 pounds; however some people may be able to lose more than that. It is most effective in the first 6 months of drug usage. It should be consumed only under prescription from a physician who will need to monitor the progress as well as track any side effects that be experienced as a result of usage of the drug. It works by reducing the absorption of fats and fat soluble vitamins A, D, E and K. Side effects include loose stools. Liver damage may also occur in some cases. It should also be avoided in case blood thinning medication is being consumed for treatment of thyroid diseases and diabetes.
2. Lorcaserin Hydrochloride can be used for weight loss for adults with BMI over 30. The consumption of the drug should be accompanied by proper dietary regulation as well as regular physical exercise. It is generally prescribed for people who have a maximum of one obesity related medical condition or disorder such as diabetes or hypertension.
3. There are certain medicines that are not FDA approved but are known to be used in the treatment of severe and morbid

obesity. These include anti-depressants, medication used to treat seizures such as zonisamide and topiramate and medicines used to treat diabetes such as metformin.

a. Certain OTC products which are not FDA approved because they are sold as dietary supplements rather than medication are utilized for achieving weight loss. These include products such as:

b. Chromium – It is an element that is used for weight loss, but correlation is not clearly established. Moreover, there are serious side effects that come along with the usage of chromium.

c. Ephedra or *ma huang* – Ephedra derived from plants contains *ephedrine* which is its active ingredient. It can lead to short term weight loss but has severe long term side effects such as increased blood pressure levels.

d. *Hoodia* cactus found in Africa is used as an appetite suppressant, and its effectiveness and safety are not known.

e. Diuretics and laxatives are commonly used for weight loss, but the weight lost is due to reduction in water and not in fat. Consumption can lead to loss of potassium in the blood and can lead to heart and muscle problems in the long run.

Surgical Procedures

In cases of morbid obesity i.e. with people having a BMI of more than 40, surgical procedures may be suggested. It may also be applicable for people with BMI greater than 35 but with a life threatening condition such as severe type 2 diabetes, cardiomyopathy and sleep apnea. Weight loss surgeries can be classified into two categories:

1. Gastroplasty – It involves using a band or even staples to create a small bag or pouch in the top section of the stomach. This essentially reduces the amount of food that the stomach is capable of holding.

2. Gastric bypass – It involves creating a bypass around a part of small intestine which is responsible for absorption of the calories. This form of surgery limits the intake of food and limits the number of calories that are absorbed by the body. There are a few side effects such as diarrhea, light headedness and nausea.

Surgeries are effective in the long run only when they are followed up with regular physical activity and balanced diet as part of a weight management program, once the weight has been brought down to manageable levels.

Weight Management – Maintenance Phase

It is one thing to lose the excess weight and another to actually maintain the new weight. For a number of people, after weight goals are achieved, relapse is quite a common occurrence and people tend to gain back all the lost weight. It is therefore extremely important to consider a weight management program as a new lifestyle rather than an object oriented short term intervention. Consuming a balanced and nutritious diet, regular physical workout and proper rest & relaxation should be incorporated and accepted as part of the new lifestyle; these have been taken up as permanent features of life, and should be enjoyed and cherished.

Body Weight Goals and How I Plan To Reach Them

Body Weight Goals and How I Plan To Reach Them

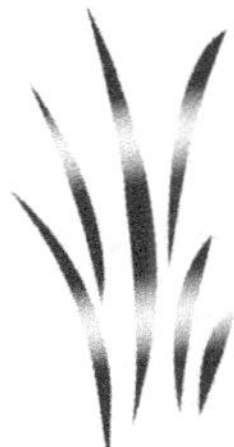

Benefits of Eating Six Small Meals A Day Versus 3 Large Meals

Understanding The Human Body

We are all aware that a weight management system plays an extremely crucial role in achieving health & fitness goals for each and every individual. Whether the goal is to lose weight or gain weight, to train for faster sprints or elite marathons, or whether it is to simply enjoy a healthy & positive lifestyle, diet and proper nutrition are cornerstones for a successful wellness plan.

Before we delve into what type of weight management plan is beneficial under what circumstances, let us first try and understand the human body and how it functions. Our body is made up of the following major components – bones, organs, fat, lean muscle tissue and water. Through a process called Body Composition Analysis we can determine the individual percentages of each of these components. Simple portable machines working on principles such as bioelectric impedance analysis and ultrasound are available which provide you the result within a few seconds. Each day newer technologies debut in the market providing more accurate results at cheaper costs. Even traditional methods such as skin-fold measurements using calipers are pretty accurate if performed properly. Understanding the body is the first step in the design of a health & fitness program, and these methods help us do this exact thing.

Out of these constituent components of the body only fat and lean muscle mass tissue are measured quantities that we aim to alter through a weight management program. If the goal is to lose weight, then we aim to reduce the amount of fat – both visceral (fat around the organs, typically the abdominal fat) & subcutaneous (under the skin, and distributed all over the body). Typically we refer to this process as healthy weight loss or fat loss. If the goal is to gain weight, then we aim to increase the amount of lean muscle mass while still maintaining or in some cases even slightly increasing the fat percentage in the body. For most people goals can be categorized into one of these two groups.

Any program that works upon changing other parameters in the body in all probability will compromise health of the individual participating in the program. For example, a weight loss gadget that gained widespread popularity was the sauna belt. As promised in all the marketing & advertising campaigns, it resulted in immediate weight loss. Within a short duration the person using the belt was able to lose weight as well as quite a few centimeters; and by short duration we mean minutes and not weeks! However, a closer inspection leads you to the crux of the functionality. It was working on dehydrating the body, essentially making you sweat and lose weight by losing water. This we can categorically state is not a healthy method to weight loss. No doubt, weight loss is achieved, but it is through dehydration and not through fat loss which is desired. Weight management plans are pretty much the most marketed products in the world each with the promise of rapid weight loss or weight gain as the case may be. However, calling a plan a product itself is the beginning of the problem. It is not something that is a one size fits all solution. Each individual is different and therefore a weight management plan has to be necessarily customized according to the specific needs of the individual.

The essential components of a weight management program aiming to achieve and maintain an optimum weight and level of health include: physical fitness, balanced & nutritious diet, adequate amount of rest and finally, mental relaxation & attitude. Each component is equally important and needs to be taken into consideration while designing a health & wellness program. In this particular section we shall be concentrating on weight management through proper nutrition.

What Do You Mean By A Weight Management Diet Plan?

The role of a good meal plan in achieving health goals cannot be over emphasized. It is one of the important pillars of a good health & wellness program. Unfortunately many people mistakenly consider it as the only pillar, convenience and control over parameter perhaps being the reasons.

A good nutritious and balanced diet goes a long way in ensuring long term good health. But what exactly do we mean by such a plan? To answer this question, we shall break up the problem into parts, starting with components of diet.

Components of Diet

Our diet is composed of hundreds of different nutrients each of them having an important function or role to play in the sustenance of a healthy life. Simply put, a nutrient is a substance in our food that provides necessary nourishment. It may help in the growth of the body, provide energy for performance of daily functions, or promote optimal health and function. Some of these nutrients are deemed essential when the body by itself is not able to provide these nutrients or is not able to provide them in sufficient quantities. We generally classify the nutrients on the basis of their function. They can be broadly categorized into the following sections:

1. Energy nutrients
    a. Carbohydrates – principal source of energy
    b. Proteins – building blocks of life, essential for tissue growth and repair
    c. Fats – energy dense molecules storing energy in the body
2. Vitamins
    a. Vitamin A, C, D, K, E, Thiamine, Riboflavin etc. – each essential for one or more of numerous biochemical reactions in the human body
3. Minerals
    a. Calcium, Iron, Zinc, Sodium, Potassium etc. – catalysts for one or more of numerous biochemical reactions taking place in the body
4. Others
    a. Water – temperature regulator as well as nutrient & hormone transport mechanism
    b. Fiber – indigestible carbohydrates playing an important role in digestion

Each of the aforementioned nutrients has multiple functions (only the most important functions have been mentioned here) and deficiency or even excess of these nutrients in the body may be harmful. It is therefore extremely important to follow a balanced diet as part of a weight management plan.

Balanced Diet

A pertinent question that arises at this stage is how we know how much of each nutrient is required by our body. The answer is given by standards such as RDA (Recommended Dietary Allowance), DRI (Dietary Reference Intakes), AI (Adequate Intake), EAR (Estimated Average Requirement) and DV (Daily Value). After extensive research across populations scientists across the world have developed these standards. They basically prescribe the quantities for intake of all these nutrients on a daily basis; variable parameters such as age and sex are taken into account. These standards themselves are not static and undergo changes on the basis of in depth research and analysis happening continuously.

A balanced weight management diet is one which provides all the nutrients in adequate quantities to maintain a balance at the same time works towards the weight goals of the program. It means that each of the specific nutrients should be consumed in quantities required to balance that which is used up by the body for the performance of daily functions as well as that which may be lost in the process. In general, non–energy nutrients such as vitamins and minerals should be consumed as per the standards prescribed. However, individuals may have variations in energy nutrients (carbohydrates, proteins & fats) depending upon their health and fitness goals. Even in these cases the meal plan should incorporate around 50 to 60% energy being provided through carbohydrates, 20 to 30% energy through fats and 15 to 20% through proteins. This ensures that while energy requirements of the body are met, simultaneously the energy nutrients are present in the correct quantities so that they are able to fulfill their other functions as well. In a nutshell the following points can be kept in mind for a balanced weight management meal plan:

1. All the micro nutrients – vitamins & minerals are consumed as per Daily Value range

2. Percentages of energy compounds – carbohydrate, protein and fat are as per suggested range
3. Adequate amount of water should be consumed – approximately 2 to 3 liters per day; this may increase depending upon environmental parameters such as temperature, humidity and altitude
4. Fiber is extremely important for digestion and adequate amounts should be consumed as part of the diet plan – roughly 25 to 35 grams per day

Key Steps in The Preparation of A Diet Plan

In this section we provide a step by step set of guidelines that should be used in the preparation of a weight management meal plan.

Step 1 – Understand The Profile of the Individual

The profile of an individual is the primary element required in the preparation of the plan. The plan for a 22 year old athlete will be very different from that of a 60 year old veteran. Similarly, it will be different for an adult woman in comparison to a man. Finally, health history and profile is extremely important to capture prior to preparation of the plan. Someone with a specific condition like rheumatoid arthritis or a deficiency such as that of Vitamin A will have a drastically different plan in comparison to someone who is not affected by these conditions.

Step 2 – Understand The Health & Fitness Goals

The goal of an endurance athlete such as a long distance runner will be very different from that of a sprinter. In a similar vein, an obese individual looking to lose weight has a completely different fitness goal in comparison to a complete ectomorph trying to gain weight. Diet plan for these individuals will be very different owing to their varied fitness goals.

Step 3 – Understand The Dietary Preferences and Lifestyle Pattern

A perfect weight management meal plan is of no use in case the individual for whom it was prepared is not able to follow it. In case a vegan is prescribed a plan wherein protein requirements are met through meat products, it is highly improbable that the plan will be successful. Not only is the content of the plan important but also the extent to which it can be followed. A plan is doomed to fail in case it demands an individual to make certain lifestyle changes that may not be possible to incorporate. For example, a person working in an organization has late working hours and goes to sleep at 3:00 am. The diet plan prescribes a meal at say 5:00 am in the morning; it is unlikely that the person will change his current job and profile for the sake of such a rigid plan.

Step 4 – Calculate The Caloric Requirement

This is the step where the mathematical calculations begin. Despite whatever scientific studies get published every day, there is one basic rule that cannot be violated. It is a natural extension from the law of conservation of energy.

IF *Energy Input* > *Energy Output* THEN *result will be Weight Gain*

IF *Energy Input* < *Energy Output* THEN *result will be Weight Loss*

By energy output we mean the total energy that the body burns during the entire day. This is a summation of the following parameters:

1. Resting Metabolic Rate (RMR) – is the total energy that the body burns in a state of complete rest. This energy is required for essential body functions, like respiration.
2. Cost of activity (COA) – is the energy that the body burns due to daily routine activities. A software professional will be burning far fewer calories during work in comparison to a manager supervising an oil rig.
3. Cost of exercise (COE) – is the total energy expended in physical workouts and exercises. A 60 year old leading a sedentary lifestyle performing limited physical exercise such as walking for half an hour burns fewer calories in comparison to a 25 year old running regularly for an hour each day.
4. Thermic effect of food (TEF) – is the energy required for digestion. A meal comprising of a high percentage of protein will require more energy to digest in comparison to a meal rich in fat or simple carbohydrates.

There are a few other parameters such as active and adaptive thermogenesis which have a relatively small contribution and are difficult to calculate. The net sum of these parameters is the total energy expended during the day and is the measure of Energy Output.

By energy input we mean the energy released in the body as a result of metabolism of food. The input depends on 2 parameters – firstly, what we eat and secondly, how much we eat. In the previous section we had discussed different energy nutrients. Each molecule of these nutrients provides exact number of calories:

1. 1 gram of Carbohydrate gives 4 calories
2. 1 gram of Protein gives 4 calories
3. 1 gram of Fat gives 9 calories
4. 1 gram of Alcohol gives 7 calories (generally kept out of consideration)

As can be expected, a gram of fat provides more than double the energy that is provided by a gram of protein or carbohydrate. Therefore, greater the percentage of energy nutrients within the meal greater will be the calorie content.

The difference between the energy input and energy output is called energy excess or deficit as the case may be. Now, to calculate the calorie requirement, we need to first understand that 1 pound of fat is roughly equivalent to 3,500 calories. Therefore, to gain or lose 1 pound of fat we need to achieve an excess or deficit of 3,500 calories. As is evident, this may be done over any length of time. For healthy weight gain or weight loss, it is suggested that the body should not undergo more than 2 pounds of change, thus ensuring that drastic and sudden changes are avoided. This is essential not only from a physical point of view but a hormonal point of view as well.

In case we want to lose 1 pound of fat on a weekly basis, then on a daily basis we need to create a deficit of approximately 500 calories. By doing our calculations, if we find that the daily energy output is 2,000 calories, then the diet within the weight management system should be made such that it provides 1,500 calories as input. By applying this process, we are able to arrive at the exact calorie requirement from the meal plan.

Step 5 – Finalize The Frequency and Timing of The Meals

The timing of meals should be such that it takes into account the following parameters:

1. Time of getting up
2. Time of going to sleep
3. Time of workout/exercise
4. Other specific times that cannot be altered for weight management plan adherence

Barring a few manageable changes, not much should be expected to be altered in the lifestyle of the person for whom the plan is being made. At the initial stage at least, this method will increase the chances of adherence. Pre-workout and post-workout meals play an extremely crucial role in deciding what energy substrate is being utilized for meeting the increased energy demands. Moreover, they also determine whether stored energy is being utilized for the purpose or the immediate input is being utilized for providing the energy. The decision is directly derived from the goals of the program and therefore it is imperative that all the steps are followed in the preparation of the diet plan. The frequency of the meals in the weight management plan is discussed in detail in the next section.

Step 6 – Design A Balanced Diet Meeting The Above Requirements

Once we have calculated the energy requirements and have arrived at the frequency and timings of the meals, the diet plan can be populated. Nutritional information regarding generic products such as whole grains and vegetables are readily available in published resources. For off the shelf products, all the information is clearly available in the nutrition data, providing which has been made mandatory. A certain amount of mixing and matching is required and at the end of this iterative process we arrive at a plan that meets all the requirements.

6 Small Meals Versus A 3 Meal Plan

Once we have understood the basic concepts of a balanced diet within the structure of a weight management system, we can now analyze in detail the pros and cons of meal plans of varying frequency.

In general, we can divide meal plans into two categories – high frequency small meal plan and low frequency large meal plan.

Since childhood during the formative years, we had been put in the habit of eating 3 meals on a daily basis – breakfast, lunch and dinner. On some days a snack may have been added here and there but this had been the pattern for numerous years. Breakfast usually meant consuming something small but energy rich, something readily available or something that could be prepared quickly. Lunch was always something that could be munched upon on the go, while dinner was the defining family meal, when everyone could sit down together after a hard day's work. Naturally this was the most enjoyable meal and perhaps the heaviest meal of the day. This matched not only our lifestyle but also that of other members of the family. The three square meals were ingrained as a concept in our dietary patterns.

However, the concept of high frequency small meals is catching up. There is no specific magic number but a 6 meal plan fits in well in our daily routine. That does not mean that a 5 meal or a 7 meal plan cannot be followed. The emphasis is on smaller meals taken more number of times during the day in a manner such that the gap between the traditional 3 meals – breakfast, lunch and dinner can be cut down.

Composition of 6 Meal Plan

Following all the steps as part of designing a healthy & balanced weight management meal plan, a generic 6 meal plan can be as following:

Meal 1 – Breakfast – As the name suggests it is the meal that literally 'breaks a fast'. It is the most important meal of the day and should comprise high energy foods to provide that energy punch required after a gap of almost 8 hours since the previous meal. A healthy mix of complex carbohydrates (those which release energy slowly over a period of time), healthy fat and proteins along with a vitamin & mineral boost through a fruit salad is ideal. Not only will such a meal be balanced in most regards, but will also provide the necessary energy required during the initial half of the day.

Meal 2 – Mid morning snack – It is essentially a snack the purpose of which is to reduce the gap between breakfast and lunch. This can simply be slices of carrot along with a nice low fat dip as accompaniment. The purpose is to cut out the gap and therefore the ensuing hunger pangs that may lead to overeating during lunch.

Meal 3 – Lunch – The afternoon meal should be well balanced comprising all essential macro nutrients as well as predominant set of micro nutrients. Ample nourishment along with appropriate energy through complex carbohydrates is the goal of this meal. Lean protein source such as grilled chicken, a decent serving of brown rice along with a bowl of vegetable salad dressed with olive oil is a good combination.

Meal 4 – Late afternoon/Evening snack – Like meal 2 it bridges the gap between lunch and dinner. Meal content is similar and can also consist of some dry fruits such as almonds along with low fat cheese or yogurt.

Meal 5 – Pre/Post workout snack – Timing of this meal is dependent on workout timings around which timings of other meals can be shuffled. Meal content is also dependent on health & fitness goals. It can include fruit/vegetable smoothies along with a protein shake. In a nutshell, in case goal is to lose fat simple carbohydrates can be cut out to a certain extent in a manner such that the body gets enough energy but at the same time gets this energy through energy substrates stored in the body such as fat and glycogen. On the other hand, if increase in lean muscle tissue is the goal, it is important to provide an insulin spike during the anabolic window immediately post workout. Therefore, a combination of simple sugars to create the insulin spike and fast acting proteins such as whey should do the trick.

Meal 6 – Dinner – On similar lines as lunch, it should be well balanced providing nourishment. However, the carbohydrate intake can be restricted since, metabolism as well as energy requirements are at a decline. It is important to also ensure that there is a small gap before pushing off to sleep. Lean protein like grilled fish, a baked vegetable preparation with sauce is a decent option.

It is important to note that there is no magic number as discussed earlier. If possible, a couple of meals such as a small pre–dinner snack to avoid hunger pangs can be incorporated within the existing structure. However, enough care should be taken so that the suggested calorie requirement is not violated at any cost. An important disclaimer here is that this is a very general plan and may not necessarily apply to specific conditions and requirements. As has been mentioned earlier a good weight management meal plan is one which is customized and tailor made suited to the goals of the individual.

Benefits of 6 Meal Plan Over A 3 Meal Plan

There are numerous benefits that are derived from breaking down 3 heavy meals into 6 lighter meals.

1. *Energy requirement matching* – The body does not require energy according to when we eat; rather we should eat to match the varying rate at which the body demands energy. Unless demanding activities like exercise routine is performed the body does not need energy in discrete shots. By breaking the heavy meals into smaller portions we provide energy to the body in a continuous manner, slowly and gradually. As can be expected, the excess carbohydrate gets converted to fat and gets stored in the body. Therefore, smaller meals are better at matching this energy requirement.
2. *Prevention of insulin spikes* – Whenever there is an increase in the level of circulating glucose in the blood stream as a result of a heavy meal, the pancreas releases insulin which then promotes the movement of this glucose into the cells, both muscle and fat cells. All cells in take up glucose from the blood to meet varied energy demands. Immediately after a meal though the fat, liver and muscle cells take up more than they require so that insulin levels can drop back to normal levels. When a heavy meal is consumed insulin spike stays on for longer resulting in storage of carbohydrates. Initially this is stored in the form of glycogen (a long chain glucose molecule) but due to limited storage capacity, excess amount starts getting converted into fat. To prevent this conversion from happening lighter meals are preferred; since calorie requirements are still to be met, greater will be the desired number of meals during the day.
3. *Promotion of utilization of stored energy reserves* – The body stores energy in the form of glucose in the blood, glycogen in the liver & muscles and finally fat in the fat cells. Whenever, energy is required it is met from either of these sources.

Insulin as described above helps and promotes the cells to utilize the carbohydrate received from the meal. Whenever extra carbohydrates enter the body through a heavy meal, the body stops depending on fat reserves stored in the body for energy production. Moreover, the extra carbohydrate again gets converted into fat. Not only is the body storing extra fat, it is also depending lesser and lesser on already stored fat in the body. This is another important factor that highlights the importance of the 6 meal plan.

4. *Prevention of sluggishness post heavy meals* – A common experience after a heavy meal is the ensuing sluggishness. The main reason for this is that to digest the large quantities of food the body is made to work that much harder. By switching to smaller meals these peaks and troughs are avoided.

5. *Decreases craving and unplanned eating* – By cutting out the large time gaps between the meals cravings that arise due to calorie controlled meals are prevented. Moreover, unplanned eating is avoided since eating a healthy snack is any which ways a part of the diet plan. Thus, by design themselves, 6 meal plans increase the chances of complete adherence to the weight management program.

6. *Prevents overeating during main meals* – In continuation with the previous benefit, uncontrolled hunger pangs that may lead to overeating during main meals are avoided. By having a small salad or vegetable smoothie prior to main meal we can prevent uncontrolled eating that may happen in case there is a long gap after the previous meal. We are then in a position to enjoy healthier options as planned.

7. *Increased metabolism* – It is commonly believed that more frequent meals help increase the metabolism rate. Whenever, meals are skipped or there is a huge time gap between meals, the body tends to go into a kind of starvation mode, thereby reducing the rate at which it uses up stored energy reserves of the body. Frequent meals specifically those rich in proteins require energy for digestion. This is where thermic effect of food also comes into play, which is the work being done by the body during this entire process. Increased metabolism will help burn the extra fat reserves stored in the body. An important disclaimer here is that this phenomenon of

increased metabolism is something that does not have a very concrete scientific base. The theory is based on the empirical studies conducted on a limited sample size. On the contrary, some researchers believe that the only way in which the metabolic rate of the body can be altered is through an increase or decrease in lean muscle tissue. Through regular exercise specifically resistance training, lean muscle tissue increases which requires energy to maintain. An increase of 1 pound of lean muscle tissue can increase the metabolic rate by up to 60 calories. Thus exercising regularly is a sure shot method to increase metabolism, and therefore should supplement the diet within a weight management program.

8. *Lower levels of LDL cholesterol* – Like in the case of metabolism, only empirical studies have shown lowering effects of 6 meal plans on LDL cholesterol, considered the bad cholesterol. The study was conducted on two sample groups, one on a 6 meal plan and the other group on a 3 meal plan. At the end of it, the 6 meal group showed significantly lower LDL cholesterol levels.

Summarizing the aforementioned points, small but frequent meals such as that proposed by 6 meal plans, help in reducing body fat percentages. Whether the goal is to gain weight or to reduce weight, a reduction of stored fat in the body is desired in most cases. This is precisely what these meal plans help in achieving.

Caveats of 6 Meal Plans That Need To Be Addressed

Despite all the benefits provided by 6 meal plans, it is important to take care of a few important points while implementing such a diet plan.

1. *Meeting calorie goals* – Whether it is a 6 meal plan or a 3 meal plan, energy excess will lead to weight gain and an energy deficit will lead to weight loss. This is the inviolable rule that overrides everything. For an individual aiming to lose weight, not only is consuming more calories than planned counterproductive to the program, consuming much lesser calories than planned can not only result in increasing body fat, it may also be harmful in the long

run. There is a possibility that during fasting this may occur with people with high fat percentages and lower activity levels.

2. *Lack of dietary control* – Some people find it extremely difficult to stop eating once they start to. For such people, a 6 meal plan may not be ideal, since they have a tendency to overeat during each of the meals. Consequently, at the end of the day, the number of calories consumed will be far greater than planned. This will lead to an energy excess and therefore weight gain. The entire purpose of the meal plan thus gets thwarted. Psychological experts propose that people who face such problems should take small but disciplined steps initially and then over a period of time embark on stricter and more rigorous plans.
3. *Customize implementation of plan* – It may not be feasible for everyone to follow such a plan to the word. It is better to take a few steps in the right direction than not move at all. For example, it may not be possible for a working professional to prepare and carry separate meals as per the 6 meal plan. In such a situation, even a meal split into two parts plays a good enough part. Improvise and customize the program but adhere to it once it has been planned.
4. *Ensure balanced diet* – At times it may happen that to ensure smaller quantity meals as part of the 6 meal plan, adequate attention may not be paid to ensure a balanced diet. Some important nutrient may get left out on a perennial basis as a result of this. Deficiency may consequently arise, which is absolutely undesirable.

On the whole, the benefits derived from small but high frequency meal plan are significant. It is not something that is only restricted to specific fitness & health goals. As a generic meal program structure it is highly advisable. The key is to ensure that it is followed in entirety and not in components. As is always the case, adherence to the plan defines the results that may be achieved through it. Inherently '6 meal plans' have a structure that promotes active adherence and make it easier for an individual to follow, thereby leading to long term health & wellness.

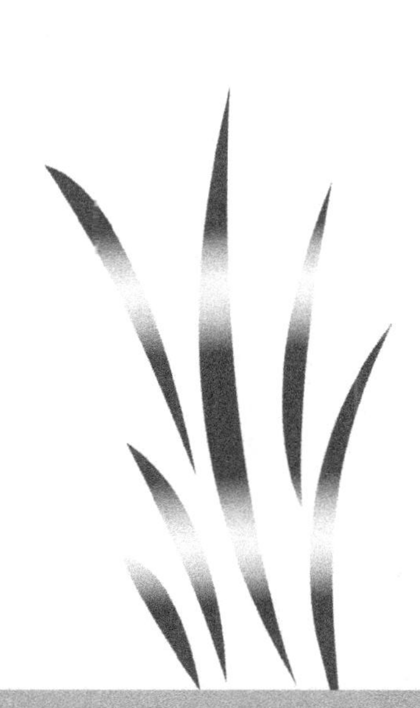

Current Eating Habits

Current Eating Habits

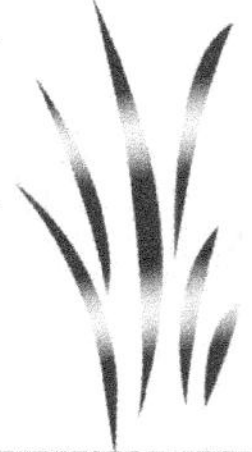

Meditation – Meaning, Types, Benefits and Impact on Weight Loss

Etymology and Meaning

Meditation is derived from the Latin verb *"meditari"* which means to think or ponder. This can further be traced back to the Hebrew language, the translation of the Hebrew Bible into Greek, led to the transformation of the root *hāgâ* into *"Melete"* (meaning *"to sigh or murmur"* and also *"to meditate")*. The Latin Bible in turned translated this root into the word on" by the Latin Bible.

A variety of words have been used to refer to "meditation" across languages and cultures e.g. the Tibetan word meditation is *"Gom"* meaning to become *"familiar with"*. This can be interpreted as familiarity to concepts positive and advantageous to our daily lives e.g. absence of fear and desire, kindness and consideration to others, tolerance, persistence etc

In modern day colloquial usage, meditation refers to the process of quiet contemplation and reflection, a process of calming the mind in order to help reduce the stress and anxiety of daily life. Sometimes it can also be linked to religion and prayer. However, to brand it in such a narrow box would be incorrect. The origin and use of mediation has spanned many centuries, across civilizations (including pre-historic), religions (Hinduism, Buddhism, Jewish, Christianity) and cultures (from India, China and Japan in the East to Europe and US in the West). In each of these the meaning and usage has taken on different nuances and meanings from an aid to peace of mind, path towards spirituality and god to a process for achievement of specific goals like concentration, compassion, detachment towards the daily life. This can also include performance of specific activities like breathing exercises, single point concentration exercises, chanting etc

The process of achieving the above can also differ from culture to religion. In some the cultures, meditation is done by being detached and cut-off from the external world and surroundings, the person having to delve within. In other forms of practice it requires the person to interact with the outside world; walking, talking, eating etc.

To summarize, there are many ways and approaches to meditation and generalizing it in a narrow definition would not be correct (similar to calling the varied art forms like writing, painting, dancing etc as the same)

History and Root

Although data suggests that some form of mediation was practiced among pre-historic civilizations (in form of chanting), written records can be traced back to 1500 BCE in Ancient India in the Vedas. In the Hindu Vedic texts it was referred to as Dhyana which comes from the Sanskrit root "*Dhyai*" meaning concentration or contemplation. Over the centuries the practice spread or developed across other countries and cultures. Although there is no clear record of the same, it is believed that the practice of meditation spread across the Eastern world around 1000 years before it spread to and gained popularity in the West.

The Buddha is known to have gained enlightenment around 500BC by sitting under the famous Banyan tree; this led to the birth of Buddhism and the Buddhist form of meditation. The text "*Pali Canon*" (a form of Buddhist scriptures) mentions meditation as a path to salvation. The silk route trade opened the doors for transmission of both Buddhism and Buddhist meditation to the other Asian countries. Over time other forms of meditation developed, Taosim in China around 5 BCE, Zen in Japan (the first meditation hall was opened in Nara, Japan in 653)

Islamic culture was also not immune to the advances of meditation, "*Dhikr*"the Islamic devotional practice of the silent recitation of the 99 names of gods can be considered a form of prayer and meditation (started around 8th / 9th century onwards). Over time Sufism (another religious practice in the Islamic word) stared to include breathing controls and repetition of words.

In western civilization, some form of meditation appears to have been mentioned around 20BCE in Greece. The writings of Philo of Alexandria hint at activities focused on attaining spirituality and aiding concentration. Around the 3rd century Plotinus had developed practices for performing meditation

Western Christian meditation developed around 6th century among monks from their practice of divine or Bible reading. Christian meditation differed from other forms in the method of its practice. As opposed to chanting / repetition of phrases, Christian meditation propagated the four formal steps of reading, pondering, praying and contemplating. In the west meditation remained in the domain of the intellectuals and saints till about the middle of the 20th century wherein it started gaining popularity among the masses as they realized the healing benefits in relieving stress, aiding relaxation and overall spiritual development.

It can be said the transmission of the knowledge about meditation came a full circle around the 1950s as a more Western and non religious form of meditation was initiated in India from the West. This then again travelled forward to the United States and Europe in the 1960s and is very similar to the more popular form of meditations as known today. This form doesn't emphasize the religious and spiritual angle of meditative techniques but focuses more on battling modern day evils like stress, and anxiety. Over time the practice of meditation has become popular enough to excite scientific curiosity also, with scientific research being performed on it in the 1970s and 1980s. However, given the various non quantifiable aspects of meditation, these studies have yet to come out with clear answers on how meditation actually works

Meditation can now truly be called a widespread and global practice with some form or the other being practices across cultures, religions and countries. In all of the above it has taken on a different mode and form, in many cases very different from the source from where it was introduced. The fact that there is no one all encompassing definition to include all the practices and desired objectives could be one of the reasons why scientists have struggled to come to any conclusive research on meditation.

Types of Meditation

Just as one size of clothes cannot fit all, in a similar manner there is no one form of meditation which can be applicable everyone.

Meditation has developed across many centuries, culture and countries. This has led to the development of many diverse forms of meditation with their own distinct practices and results. Which particular form is suitable to an individual can depend upon factors like personality, state of mind at the point, external surroundings etc. They key is to choose the technique with which the person is most comfortable with rather than what is considered the "in thing" at the moment.

There is no single authority / text which can be conclusively referred to for providing detailed information on the various types of meditation. However, over the years certain distinctive techniques have developed which have come to be popularly accepted as separate types. Most of them have the flow of breath as a common linking factor. While some techniques give more importance to breathing (making the inhaling and exhaling as a focal point of the technique), others make it as one of the factors to be noticed while practicing. It is not possible to provide an exhaustive list of all of the meditation techniques being practiced around the world, given their sheer number, however below we give some of the major types being practiced.

The list below lists the different types of meditation forms being practiced based on the technique, however this can also be done on the basis of the religion (e.g. meditation in Buddhism, Christianity, Hinduism, Jainism, Islam etc). Given how meditation techniques have travelled across the world, many of the above religions would have similar techniques being used.

Mindfulness Meditation

It is one of the most popular types of meditation, especially in the West. As the name suggests, it is a meditation in which one is aware of one's surroundings and does not endeavor to block out the external world and associated sounds. The idea is to let the thoughts flow through your mind but without becoming attached or focused on any particular thought. This does not necessarily require quite surroundings (though they may be useful), this can be performed in the middle of a crowded park with people all around also. The aim would be to let all the sounds just flow thorough mind in a detached manner. Some people also refer to this process as "*Vipassana*". Breathing while important (as in most types of meditation) is not a key element here. It is one of the many thoughts and flows which go through the mind

In practice, mindfulness meditation can be useful for beginners. They are more likely to find it difficult to empty the mind and focus on nothingness and perform other more technical forms of meditation. The lack of attachment to any particular thought is what aids in relaxation of the individual.

Focused Meditation

This is the next step in taking up for advanced meditation techniques. It involves focus on a particular thought throughout the entire process. The thought can be something internal (like imagining a particular object or situation) as well as external (like a sound or a chant). The thought in itself is not important, the unwavering focus on the thought is.

Given the broad scope of the above type, there are a few offshoots to focused meditation

- Guided Visualization – This refers to focused meditation on some thought or imaginary situation. In popular usage instructors / guides asks their students to imagine their special comfort place. Some kind of external recordings can also be played to aid the imagination e.g. playing the sound of leaves rustling to facilitate thoughts of a jungle or wooded field.
- Rhythm Based Meditation - This involves focus on any bodily rhythm e.g. breathing or beating of the heart. The idea is that by giving full focus / attention to any particular rhythm, other thoughts are more likely to melt away and not disturb the mental peace. Thus a practitioner will be focusing on each inhale and exhale, controlling his / her breaths by making them deeper, slower and fuller which would prevent the mind from wandering on other external thoughts.

Mantra Meditation

In Hindu texts and philosophy it is believed that certain words provide a positive vibration when chanted or spoken out loudly. These can referred to as Mantras, for example the syllable *"Om"* (pronounced as AUM) when chanted out aloud is supposed to have many healing benefits and is used in religious ceremonies in India. Mantra meditation combines the benefits of meditations and these positive vibrations. The chanting also helps the practitioner to focus his mind and empty it of other thoughts.

In more advanced forms Mantra Meditation can be called as **Transcendental Meditation**. It emerges from the Hindu form of meditation, and while it is practiced by the chanting of a Mantra the focus is on becoming detached from all that is materialistic and transient. A practitioner in the more advanced stages of Transcendental Meditation will focus on altering the breath to actually change the state of existence with the ultimate aim of leaving the materialistic body behind (also referred to as *"Samadhi"* in India)

Kundalini Meditation

This is another form of meditation which has roots in Vedas in the Hindu culture. It is based on the concept that all human beings have a certain number of energy centers in their bodies with one being on top of the head also. Energy in our body is moves in an upward moving stream to this energy center on top of the head and from their into infinity (in some cases it can be considered moving into the ultimate energy source of all universe). The idea behind the meditation is to move with this rising stream of energy upwards into perpetuity. As opposed to some of the other techniques described above, this form of meditation focuses on breathing and makes it a key factor in its implementation. The meditation practitioner is supposed to concentrate on the flow of breath through each of the energy centers and finally into breathing. The focus on any one activity being performed in the body also helps to empty the mind of other unwanted thoughts.

Qi Gong Meditation

Qi Gong Meditation derives from the Taoist form of meditation where breathing is the focus of the practitioner. Similar to Kundalini meditation this form also believes in energy centers in the body and the flow of energy through them. However, in this form there are three major energy centers; forehead center, chest center and two inches below the navel. The focus is on flow of energy (via breathing) through the various organs and energy centers, but in an oval manner referred to as the *"microcosmic orbit"* (like an energy channel encircling the upper part of the body). This process of energy circulation is called as *"Qi"* or *"Chi"*. This flow of energy is supposed to improve blood circulation thereby improving the brain function by increase in secretion of some vital chemicals.

Zazen Meditation

Zazen refers to the Japanese Buddhist form of meditation. It is a more advanced form of meditation as it provides minimal guidance on how it has to be learnt and performed. It is generally done for extended time periods and only basic instructions with respect to the posture are given (sitting with a straight back). Although there is no particular focus on breathing, it can be done in combination with focus on some Buddhist scripture. Given the minimalistic approach towards instruction, it is more suited individuals in a more simple and Spartan surroundings.

Spiritual Meditation

This form of meditation is more entwined with religion as compared to others described above. It is a meditation more suited for those who anyways offer prayer on a regular basis as it is based on interaction and communication with god and the spirit world. The idea behind this technique is to empty your mind of external thoughts, become relaxed, calm and detached from the outer world and then try and feel the oneness with the spiritual forces in the world. Focusing on breathing can be a good way to start so quiet the mind, once that has been achieved the mind is more free to explore the link between the conscious and sub conscious world.

Trance Based Meditation

This can be considered a more advance form of Spiritual Meditation. In some spheres this is not considered a proper form of meditation as there is a lack of self control and can at times involves the usage of intoxicants or hypnotism to produce the trance like state. This form of mediation is characterized by an absence of control, rational thinking and the feeling of no longer being part of the body. If this effect has been produced by external stimulus (hypnotism or intoxicants) then memory of experiencing this mediation can be limited for the practitioner. This can be a negating factor at times because without knowledge of the control gained over the mind, the use in daily life can be limited. Apart from intoxicants and hypnotism music and even rapid breathing can be used to induce this state.

Movement Meditation

As the name suggests, unlike all of the above forms of meditation, under this technique the practitioner has to move to meditate. There are no fixed movements to perform this; they can be slow and rhythmic like the gentle swaying of the body, hands, head, etc, the gentle movements helping to calm the mind. They can also be fast and intense movements to breakthrough some stubborn thoughts and molds in our thoughts and body, post which a more calming state can be achieved. The practice of *"Osho"*, which has gained a lot of popularity over the last few years draws heavily from this form of meditation.

While the above forms and techniques outline some of the more popular forms of meditation being practiced today, it is virtually impossible to compile and exhaustive list given the many offshoots of each of the above techniques which exist and are being created even as we speak. Different cultures adopt a particular kind of technique and then adapt it to their own surroundings to create a new form of meditation.

Benefits of Meditation

Meditation is not an exact science. While over the past many years there has been an increase in scientific interest in meditation and its many benefits, there have been no conclusive or authoritative results on what meditation is, how it works and what are its benefits. However, having said that, there are many benefits (and even miracles) which have been attributed to meditation over the centuries. These range from the physical to the metaphysical. Broadly speaking, the benefits of meditation can be broken down into three broad categories Physical or Health Related, Mental or Psychological and Spiritual

Physical or Health Related Benefits

In modern day lifestyles stress is the cause of many of our health problems, from heart diseases to diabetes to hypertension. While meditation is not a medicine which can scientifically cure the disease itself, it helps to attack these problems at the root to prevent their occurrence and minimize the negative impact if the person is already suffering from them. Meditation can provide a two-fold benefit here. Meditative techniques provide a calming effect and help reduce stress thereby preventing the onset of the diseases and the positive energy / vibrations released help reduce the negative impact of the diseases. Meditation helps reduce the production of Cortisol (hormone associated with stress levels). Studies have shown that regular meditation helps to increase the strength of alpha waves being produced in the body, these alpha waves are associated with a peaceful and quiet state of the mind (similar to sleep). This relaxed state further inhibits the production of lactic acid in the blood associated with high anxiety levels.

Given below are some of the many health related benefits of meditation which people have experienced over the years (as stated above, these are not medically or scientifically proven benefits, but those which many people have experienced as they practiced meditation).

1. Breadth control in meditation helps to slow the body down, its heart rate and oxygen utilization rate. This helps in fighting against hypertension, blood pressure, anxiety attacks
2. Meditation is also known to strengthen the immune system which helps in fortifying the body against germs and viruses and also aids in healing (be it from the common cold to post-op recovery)
3. Meditation is known to help balance the hormonal system which can help women before and during the menstruation cycle. Hormonal balance can also help both men and women in emotional control in their daily lives.

4. Meditation can help control cholesterol levels which can help in fighting heart diseases and diabetes.
5. Meditation is also known to help control weight problems and in aiding weight loss (more details on this later).
6. Meditation overall improves the health and well-being of an individual which makes them more energetic and positive in their approach.
7. Meditation is also known to increase sperm and ovulation count in men and women, which in turn helps battle infertility. This also could be attributed to the reduction of stress and tension which is known to have a negative impact on sperm and ovulation count.
8. Meditation improves stress levels which help control anger and temper and their harmful side-effects on the human body.
9. Recent scientific studies have concluded that meditation can also transform the brain and alter brain activity. Scientific experiments conducted have shown that there was a change in the grey matter of people who were doing regular meditation. There was an increase noticed in parts of the brain responsible for memory, learning and emotional quotient and decrease in those associated with anxiety and stress

Mental or Psychological Benefits

Meditation provides a number of psychological benefits also. As mentioned above, meditation helps in the production of alpha waves which help ease anxiety and stress. Meditation slows down the frantic pace of brain activity brought out by our over-crowded lives. This does not mean that the person becomes less intelligent or capable, as the level of awareness actually improves. It just means that the person becomes calm and composed, able to view the external world in a more detached manner which helps in decision making. People who practice meditation regularly feel rejuvenated and recharged post meditation, increasing their efficiency in whatever work they choose to do. This serene and tranquil state leads to a host of benefits, some of which have been outlined below.

1. One of the most important benefits of practicing meditation is mental control. Regular practice enables the practitioner

to prevent the minds from moving from thought to thought and to focus it on a particular subject. This improves the mental sharpness, capability and concentration of a person making him / her much more efficient in any work they perform

2. Mental control also leads to control over moods and emotions. Regular practice can help control moods swings, extreme displays of negative emotions such as anger, jealousy, hate etc.

3. Increase in control not only makes a person more likable but also helps improve self confidence and self esteem.

4. Regular practice also helps a person to overcome their phobias and fears. People start seeing the phobias for what they are, imaginary situations / events / people etc which have been blown out of proportion by an overstressed and overworked mind.

5. A meditative person becomes a better listener. He / she is able to better understand what others are saying, exhibit self control in times of extreme emotional outbursts by the other, and is overall able to behave in much more healthier and mature manner. All of these help the person to form and sustain better and longer lasting relationships both in their professional and personal set up.

6. Meditation helps to calm the mind. A stressed person's brain is overloaded with multitude of thoughts, each pushing and shoving to get mind space. More likely than not such a person is likely to suffer from insomnia as some thought or the other is keeping him / her awake. Meditation helps to sort out all of these thoughts and clear the mind, leading to a healthy sleep. Such people do not have to sleep long hours also as the hours they have slept have been refreshing enough for the mind.

7. Focus and concentration make a person sharper, more alert and better able to solve react in a sudden problem situation. This improves the problem solving skills of the person.

8. A healthy mind and body leading to a happy and fulfilling life obviate the need of external stimulus or intoxicants (hypnosis, drugs, smoking, liquor etc) to help produce a happy and satisfied state. This helps to combat drug and other forms of substance abuse.

9. Meditation is also known to foster the creative aspects of the brain
10. All of the above benefits help produce a well rounded and balanced personality, able to handle a variety of situations with ease.

Spiritual Benefits

One of the biggest advantages of meditation is the spiritual aspects. Practitioners, especially regular practitioners are able to rise above their daily lives and routine and observe things from a more broader and holistic manner. It is said that human beings use just a fraction of their brains in their daily lives. Meditation helps us to harness the energy in the remaining part and develop the subconscious self. This can bring about immense change in the personality of the individual, with the chores of the daily life not seeming arduous any more, and the person becoming more involved in questions like the purpose of life itself. Some of the spiritual benefits and changes which can be observed by practicing meditation are

1. Increase in kindness and consideration towards others – One of the basic benefits of meditation is reduction in hostility towards the external environment. Meditation helps bring a peace of mind which improves acceptance of and tolerance towards others. This forms the building block, from this stems the knowledge that all of us are on the same path towards self realization, this unity of purpose in turn increases kindness and consideration towards others
2. Synchronization between the body (physical), mind (ego) and soul (spirit) – One of the biggest causes of conflict in our lives is the disagreement between the mind, body and soul. With a clash in their purposes the self gets torn between various actions (with the body and mind living more in the physical world and the soul concerned with the cosmic). Meditation reduces our dependence and desire for the physical world and helps bridge this gap.
3. Reduced emphasis on the ego- Most people are very caught up in their image of themselves. At times this desire to "be someone" becomes an obsessive force which prevents us from enjoying our lives. Meditation helps us to realize that

the physical self is a tiny part in the universe and in our wider calling providing much needed humility to our lives.

4. Acceptance, of external as well as internal events – There are many teachers who preach that the external world is an ephemeral part of our lives and there is a wider and deeper meaning to our lives. However, at times, events in this transient life can cause us much hurt and pain. These emotions stem from our non-acceptance of the events happening in our lives, a master is rarely perturbed by events around him / her. Meditation helps us gain this perspective and increases our acceptance.
5. Infinite capacity for love – Meditation provides us with a wider understanding of the world around us. It makes us realize that each individual / soul is on the path of self discovery and their acts and deeds are just an unconscious way of reaching the path. This not only makes us more forgiving towards them but the unity of our goal increases our love towards them. Meditation also makes us realize that love can answer many more questions and open many more doors than hate. We start to understand how much more true and complete joy is there in spreading love than jealousy and hatred.
6. Communion with god – All of the above take us step by step closer toward the creator. We start to realize in believe in a loving and compassionate god who is always there to help us in times of need. Regular meditation can hasten our spiritual union with god
7. Helps attain "Nirvana" or enlightenment – This is the final stage of masters and teachers. When there is realization of our true purpose on earth, when the daily lives and responsibilities are left behind for a higher calling. Meditation helps answer the question "Who am I and why am I here".

To summarize, there are multitude benefits of meditation, ranging from the physical to the spiritual. Depending upon the level of practice and expertise of the practitioner, he / she is able to move higher up the ladder and avail of more advantages. Different types of meditation listed above have different advantages and can be chosen accordingly as per the goal of the practitioner.

Meditation and Weight Loss

People always associate weight loss with proper eating and regular exercise, sitting quietly (even motionless) in place generally doesn't fall into the category of "things to do for weight loss". While meditation is less effective in actually burning the fat like a workout does, it is extremely important in creating the right kind of (internal) atmosphere needed for losing the weight. Exercise in itself can be pointless if we continue to have a negative approach or are irregular in our efforts. Below are some of the reasons why mediation is an invaluable tool to help is in shedding those extra pounds.

1. Helps identify the root of our weight problem – Without identifying the source of the weight issues, exercise and diet can often be in vain. Even if the individual is able to lose weight, it is unlikely to be permanent until the root cause has also been addressed. For example many people tend to binge eat when angry, stressed, unhappy etc. Thus no matter how hard they try, weight loss techniques are unlikely to be successful or permanent until they are able to bring some peace and calm in their life or break the vicious circle between extreme emotions, eating and weight gain.
2. Increased determination and self control – Weight loss is not just about the physical activity or restriction of calorie intake, there are many more factors at work to get that perfect figure or body. A person can have the best of intentions about losing weight, but without the mental control and determination to put these into practice, chances of success are slim. Just knowing that they have to exercise regularly and reduce high calorie food is not useful; it is the doing which is going to help achieve the results. Meditation can help bring this focus and determination. One of the many benefits of meditation is self control, focus and single-mindedness of purpose, which help in weight loss.
3. Reduces comfort eating – One of the most common reasons for gaining weight are stress and anxiety eating. Many people who find a void in their lives tend to fill it with food. This is frequently referred to as emotional eating and is not done out of a physical desire for food but emotional desire of fulfillment. Meditation helps a person focus inwards and

reduces the need for external praise and acceptance. When the sense of fulfillment is coming from within, external stimulus in the form of food is no longer required. Recent studies have indicated that even extreme positive emotions can cause excessive eating as the body is not able to distinguish between extreme positive and negative stimulus. Meditation helps to bring a more balanced approach to life and thinking which negates the impact of both extreme positive and negative reactions

4. Reduction in desire – A corollary of the above benefit is the decrease in desire itself. As has been stated above in the "Benefits of Meditation" sector, a regular practitioner rises above the chores and pressures of daily lives. He / she realizes that our physical existence is just a means to achieve a higher goal. This leads to a reduction in dependence and desire on external stimuli. Masters and ascetics have been known to survive little or no food for extended periods of time. While this is an extreme example of highly developed individuals, regular practitioners are also able to achieve a reasonable reduction in desire in their daily lives, which in turn can help in weight loss.

5. Positive thoughts/ visualization help achieve the goal – Many studies have shown that positive thinking is an essential tool in achieving any goal (whether it be a desired job, promotion or weight loss). It has been shown that a person's thoughts can be a strong force in creating his / her reality. Thus a person is imagining himself /herself to be overweight and fat, is likely to negate the positive effects of regular exercise and healthy eating. Meditation helps to control the minds and push out any negative thoughts and fears, to be replace with positive, healthy and more conducive thoughts

6. Provides a balanced approach to thinking, thereby limiting both binge eating and starvation – Meditation helps to reduce excessive emotions. A regular practitioner is less likely to be affected by both extreme positive or negative news. Studies have shown that habitual eating can at times be caused by strong emotions, thus limiting their impact on the self is likely to help in weight loss. Meditation also provides a measure of balanced thinking in life; regular practitioners are less likely

to be impatient for immediate results as they will realize that all things happen at their own time and pace. This is apt to reduce the need for severe crash diets followed by equally strong binge eating sessions as the body starts to crave food.

7. Helps control hormones associated with weight gain – Apart from the mental benefits of meditation on weight gain, it also helps by controlling the secretion of negative hormones. Studies have shown that Cortisol (hormone associated with increased stress levels) also inhibits the body's ability to fight fat deposits. Meditation helps to reduce the production Cortisol in our body which in turn helps with weight loss.

8. Helps improve "Mindfulness" – Meditation helps a person become more mindful or aware of what they are doing. Thus in the case of compulsive eaters, meditation can make them aware of why they are eating, what they are eating, how much, are they actually taking pleasure in the eating or is it just a mechanical activity being performed. This helps in reducing "habit" part of eating and replaces it with "need", thereby helping in weight loss.

There have been studies done in which groups of people have been taught meditation and given lessons on mindful eating alongside with regular meditation. Results have shown that people who were able to successfully learn mindful eating and meditation had a drop in their Cortisol levels and experienced more weight loss than the others. The weight loss can be attributed to the reduced Cortisol levels and also sensory changes in the brain associated with hunger and desire.

The purpose of the above points is not to claim that weight loss can be achieved by performing meditation alone (although such cases have also been there). The purpose is to illustrate that meditation is an extremely useful tool in the entire process of weight loss. It can speed up and improve the effectiveness of the other weight loss means being used (e.g. exercise and calorie control). By helping a person visualize himself/ herself in a more positive manner, meditation is able to harness the energy of the subconscious mind to aid in weight loss.

Goals

Goals

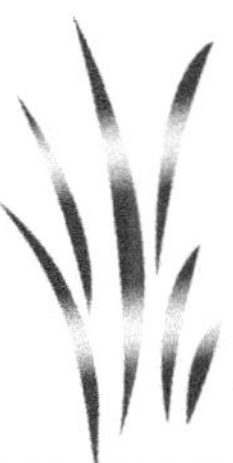

What is Yoga?

'Yoga', derived from the Sanskrit word *'yuj'* literally meaning 'to unite', is a combination of physical, mental and spiritual disciplines finding its origin in ancient India. The union referred to in the name is that of the individual with the universal spirit. It is one of the most ancient sciences and its origin is dated back to the origin of civilization itself. According to Hindu mythology, it is believed to have originated some 26,000 years ago in the age referred to as *Satyug* or the golden age; an age with an everlasting abundance of peace with people living harmoniously in their quest for the eternal truth. A few classical texts in fact propound *Lord Shiva*, the Hindu God as the first yogic teacher whereas the *Bhagwad Gita,* the holy Hindu scripture advocates *Lord Krishna* as the first teacher. The primary tools commonly used to practice yoga include physical postures or *asanas*, breathing techniques or *pranayama* and meditation or *dhyana.*

Yoga is a practical science or a discipline which is put to use to attain a specific goal. The purpose of yoga in general, is linked to the theological or philosophical school it is associated with. In some schools the purpose is devotion to take pleasure from constant experience of God, while in others it is the experience of *Brahman* or that which pervades all things. In modern times though, yoga is commonly understood as being a combination of numerous physical postures and breathing techniques that helps in elimination of various health problems and ailments, at the same time providing relaxation by alleviating stress.

We might know a bit about yoga, but to understand it in a better manner, it is important to understand the history of yoga right from the time of its origin.

Origin and History of Yoga

Until recently it was believed by numerous western scholars that yoga originated around 500 BC, which is roughly the time of the Buddha, founder of Buddhism. In the 1920's, archaeologists discovered the

Indus valley civilization. In the excavated material were several seals that depicted common yoga and meditation poses. These seals were dated to the third millennium BC. Despite the absence of concrete proof, there is a certain resemblance between the postures depicted in these excavated seals and yoga practices of a later date. The history of yoga can be classified into four categories:

Vedic Yoga

Vedas are the oldest scriptures in the world. They were composed in a very archaic version of Sanskrit and were passed on from one generation to the next only by word of mouth. Considering the massive size of the scriptures such a process seems simply unfathomable, yet it is true beyond doubt. The *Vedas* mean knowledge and were essentially a collection of hymns. The four Vedas included *rig veda (rig* meaning praise) – the foremost scripture which has references that suggest that certain components may have been composed as long ago as the third millennium BC. The other three Vedas are *yajur veda, sama veda* and *atharva veda* essentially books of songs, rituals and spells respectively. The people during this age relied upon vedic seers or *rishis* to teach them the essence of life and the concepts of divine harmony. These seers lived in seclusion in forests and were known to possess powers of intuition gained through spiritual practice. The yoga of this period was connected to ritual life. By performing specific rituals with extreme focus levels it was aimed to enjoin the material and spiritual world. Such strong focus over prolonged periods for overcoming the limitations of the mind is the essence of vedic yoga.

Pre–Classical Yoga

The pre–classical period covers a period of over 2,000 years, right until 200 AD. The yoga of this period is characterized by the Upanishads which is where the first usage of the term yoga seems to appear. There are more than 200 scriptures as part of the Upanishads which contain the essence of Vedas – ultimate unity of the entire universe is the hidden teaching. *Katha Upanishads* define yoga as the achievement of the supreme state through cessation of all mental activities. This is done through a gradual control gained over all the senses. Concepts such as *kundalini* and *chakra* (explained later) as well as the relationship between breath and thought process are mentioned in these texts. However, the goal of yoga in the Upanishads was clearly the transcendent self.

The *Bhagwad Gita* was the song of the Lord as narrated by Lord Krishna to the warrior prince Arjun. The usage of the term yoga has been done in numerous ways within the text. Apart from the traditional practice & meditation it contains information on *karma yoga* or action, *bhakti yoga* or devotion, *jnana yoga* or knowledge.

The *Mahabharata* and *Ramayana* are two of the greatest Indian epics – *Mahabharata* being the longest poem in the world (more than six times the content of Odyssey and Iliad combined). These epics contain the teachings of many schools of the era which taught the practice of deep meditation. Yogis practicing these techniques could transcend mind & body thus understanding their true spiritual essence and the unity of the one and all.

Classical Yoga

This period between 500 BC to 500 AD was the period of Mauryan and Gupta dynasties. It is during this period that different forms of yoga began to emerge in different Hindu, Buddhist and Jain philosophical schools. Classical yoga is marked by the creation of *Yoga Sutra.* It was created by Patanjali and is considered the culmination of the systematization process of yoga that had started at the beginning of this period. They were written around 200 AD and seem to have considerable influence from previous schools of the era. The Yoga Sutras are terse as well as complicated. They are often studied along with *Yoga Bhashya* which is essentially a collection of commentaries on *Yoga Sutra* written in the fifth century providing explanations to cryptic and complicated components. The form of yoga arising from *yoga sutras* is called *Raja yoga* and it emphasizes control over the mind.

The *Yoga Sutra* contains 196 *sutras* or threads divided into chapters:

1. *Samadhi Pada* which deals with the nature of *Samadhi* or perfect concentration
2. *Sadhana Pada* deals with the process of refining and cleansing the mind, body & soul

3. *Vibhuti Pada* deals with yogic properties and integration achieved through meditation. It also deals with super natural powers and gifts.
4. *Kaivalya Pada* deals in the relationship of the yogi with the soul

The *Yoga Sutras* lead to the birth of the system known as *Ashtanga Yoga* or eight–limbed form of yoga. It is the core characteristic of every form of *Raja yoga* being practiced today. The eight components are as following:

1. *Yama* means social restraints and covers the 5 abstentions – *ahimsa* or non–violence, *asteya* or non–covetousness, *brahmacharya* or celibacy, *satya* or truth and finally *aparigraha* or non–possessiveness
2. *Niyama* means observing purity & tolerance and covers the 5 observances – *shaucha* or purity, *tapas* or austerity, *santosha* or satisfaction, *svadhyaya* or study of the scriptures to understand God and finally *ishvara–pranidhana* or surrender to the almighty
3. *Asana* means seat, referring to the position for meditation but covers all the postures and physical exercises
4. *Pranayama* means breath regulation and control
5. *Pratyahara* means withdrawal of senses while preparing for meditation
6. *Dharana* means concentration and focusing attention on one specific object
7. *Dhyana* means meditation
8. *Samadhi* means ecstasy through liberation

It was believed as part of this school that individual is composed of both matter and spirit. Contrary to Vedic and pre–classical yoga, it was believed that it was essential to separate the two for attaining purity of spirit.

Post–Classical Yoga

This is the post–Patanjali period up till present date during which numerous schools have sprung up that are derived from or in some cases even independent from his work. During this period, the focus shifted to the present, and emphasis was on accepting reality and living in the present moment rather than focusing only on liberation. There was a distinct turn in attention from purely the mind & soul to the physical body. Yogis in previous eras concentrated upon the union with the universal one, however now, attention towards the body was given equal emphasis. This resulted in development of practices that rejuvenated the body in a way to promote and prolong a healthy life.

Bhakti yoga became popular as part of the *bhakti movement* in the 12th century AD. It advocated meditative practices with devotion towards God. Yogis such as *Surdasa, Meerabai* and *Tulsidasa* popularized *bhakti yoga. Hatha yoga* period started from the 9th century AD and was at its peak during the 14th century AD. It was started by *Gorakshanath* and *Matsyendranath* who were *shivaite* ascetics. It is sometimes also called psychophysical yoga because of its basis on the premise that a pure physical body will lead to a pure mind. It takes up the *asanas* from *yoga sutras* and converts them into full postures; it is these postures that are associated with yoga today. Many texts have been written during this period and different personalities came to the forefront with their schools of teaching. A few prominent ones include *Sri Shankaracharya* in the 8th century AD and *Ramanujacharya* in the 11th century AD.

Modern yoga

Modern yoga is considered to begin with the Parliament of Religions that was convened in the year 1893 in Chicago. In this convention *Swami Vivekanand* created a lasting impression in the minds of the audience. He was the first person to disseminate and promote various aspects of yoga to the western world during his tours to the US and Europe. In continuation with the gradual introduction of physical aspects of yoga in the previous era, modern yoga is also associated with *asanas* as a form of exercise. Gradually yoga has been able to shed its connection with purely religious contexts, making it generally more acceptable to world audience. Over the years, the health benefits from regular practice of yoga has been documented and published widely. As a result of which more 20 million people practice yoga in the US alone.

Different Types of Yoga

Since the classical period numerous forms of yoga have been taught by various schools. Each of them has different driving philosophies as well as distinct methods of practice.

1. *Raja yoga* – It refers to the system advocated by Patanjali in *Yoga Sutra*. The eight limb system described in the previous section forms the basis of *raja yoga.* It is a form which is practiced by refinement of behavior through restraint, discipline, physical health through postures, breathing techniques, sensory withdrawal, concentration, meditation and finally liberation.
2. *Hatha yoga* – *Hatha yoga* is based on the book called *Hatha yoga pradipika* written around the 12th century AD by *Swami Swatmarama.* It is a systematic combination of techniques aimed at cleansing of mind & body and effects consciousness. It is a combination of *asanas* or practice of full body postures, *pranayama* or breathing techniques, *mudras* or gestures signifying mental attitudes, *bandhas* or energy locks, *nada* or sound and meditation. It is one of the most commonly practiced forms of yoga and is generally associated as representative of yoga for most people. It is believed that if practiced in the right manner it not only helps in getting rid of various mental and physical ailments but also increases the *pranic energy* leading to stability, sound health as well as lightness of body & mind.
3. *Mantra yoga* – *Mantras* are essentially verses from the Vedas. This school of yoga believed that the chanting of these *mantras* will lead to salvation or union with the one. The bottom line though is that one needs to have complete and unconditional faith in the power of the *mantra* without which it will simply be recitation, which will simply be futile. *Mantras* are generally classified into 2 categories – *tantric* (originated from the *tantras* and practiced for certain specific purposes) and *puranic* (relatively simple form that can be easily learnt and practiced). The selection of the *mantra* or verse can be done by the Guru (also called *guru mantra*), it could be the *universal mantra or Om,* it could even be based on the basic inherent nature of the individual (different mantras such as *gayatri mantra*

and *mahamrutyunjay mantra* suit different natures of individuals)

4. *Bhakti yoga* – *Bhakti* or complete devotion to God is the basis of this form of yoga. The concept of personal God also came into picture during the *bhakti movement*. The universal supreme is manifested in various forms, be it Krishna, Rama, Buddha or Jesus. This form of yoga works by the process of channelizing the emotional energy towards the object of devotion. Suppressed emotions in the individual are considered to be the reason behind all forms of physical as well as mental ailments, through *bhakti yoga* these suppressed emotions get released leading to purification of mind & body.
5. *Karma yoga* – *Karma* literally means work in Sanskrit and this form of yoga emphasizes complete devotion to work as the path to salvation. Whenever a person does some work there is an outcome or an end to which the person starts getting attached to. In the practice of *karma yoga* this attachment is what one aims to cut out so that selfless work is what remains. In this state the mind becomes stable and is not affected by the ups & downs that are associated with the output of what work one does. In this state of mind work comes to represent devotion and it should therefore be practiced without attachment of any kind to the end result.
6. *Jnana yoga* –In Sanskrit *Jnana* literally means knowledge, but in the current context it means wisdom attained through self awareness. Through a process of meditation it is possible to attain wisdom and understand true nature of inner knowledge. Self realization is the goal that is sought through meditation.
7. *Kundalini yoga* – There are psychic *chakras* that are believed to exist in each and every individual. The 6 main chakras include *mooladhara* or coccygeal, *swadishtana* or sacral, *manipura* or solar, *anahata* or cardiac, *vishuddhi* or cervical, *ajna* or pineal, *bindu and sahasrara* or cerebellum. Through the practice of this form of yoga the goal is to awaken these various *chakras* or psychic centers. There are different layers of the mind, each associated with a particular level of consciousness and different *chakras.* Through

kundalini yoga a yogi tries to awaken the higher level *chakras* through deep concentration that then forces their arousal. The awakening can be stimulated by a combination of *asanas, pranayama, mudras and bandhas*. Even other forms of yoga such as *mantra yoga* can be utilized to cause the awakening.

8. *Swara yoga – Swara* in Sanskrit means note or sound. It also represents the flow of air through the nostrils. Thus this form of yoga aims at union through the manipulation and control of breath. Whereas *pranayama* relates only to the ways in which breath can be controlled and is basically a group of breathing techniques, *swara yoga* also incorporates observation and study of breath apart from manipulation and control. Therefore it more comprehensive in nature.

Apart from these, there have been numerous schools that have sprung up of late, specifically in the 19th and 20th century AD. Quite a few of them have gained popularity in the west. These schools have been able to translate complicated ritualistic forms of yoga to simpler forms which can be practiced by a layman. By their emphasis on the health benefits derived from regular practice of yoga these schools have been able to engage the attention of the masses by their emphasis on present world real life. A few forms that have gained quite a bit of prominence of late include the following:

1. *Anusara yoga* is one of the relatively newer forms of yoga started in 1997, which is a combination of difficult postures but emphasizes the playful spirit and opening up of the heart while still performing the *asanas* with correct alignment.
2. *Bikram Yoga* was started by Bikram Choudhury and is based on the belief of a comprehensive workout that includes muscular strength, cardiovascular endurance, muscular endurance and flexibility. Unique about this form of yoga is that it is practiced in a heated environment usually at 95 to 105 degrees Fahrenheit. It is believed that in such an environment yoga promotes detoxification.
3. *Iyengar Yoga* is one of the most popular forms of yoga and was developed by B.K.S.Iyengar in the 1970's. It is a form of *hatha yoga* that uses different types of props such as cushions, blocks and belts that helps even the elderly and disabled to perform the

asanas. These *asanas* are generally held for longer periods of time, a minute or so or may be even more. The slow movements along with usage of props that enable everyone to participate have made this form of yoga extremely popular.

4. *Power Yoga* is the modern version of *ashtanga yoga*, an American interpretation that includes most of the *asanas* being performed with vigor. The *asanas* resemble callisthenic workouts such as toe touches, push-ups and head stands. It lays emphasis on moving from one *asana* to another without any rest. Such fast paced continuous aerobic activity leads to burning fat and consequently healthy weight loss

These newer forms of yoga have adapted themselves in a manner to appeal to the masses and make yoga accessible to everyone. Maintaining the basic premises of traditional yoga forms, these new schools add variety in a manner that they provide a holistic workout to the person practicing yoga. Gradually emphasis has shifted from yoga being a spiritual study to it becoming a practice for achieving and maintaining a healthy body and a calm and peaceful mind.

Benefits of Yoga

It is commonly believed that practicing yoga on a regular basis increases flexibility and promotes balance and coordination. However, this is a myopic viewpoint because most people understand yoga as a combination of *asanas* or body postures. Yoga practiced in its entirety not only has physiological benefits but also has a tremendous positive impact on the psychological and spiritual fronts of life.

Physiological Benefits

1. Flexibility – The various *asanas* or postures help in stretching various muscles of the body. These postures are very similar to static stretches that are performed slowly and in which position is held for a brief period of time. Often people feel they are too stiff or old to perform yoga; on the contrary yoga is for everyone. Slow, controlled movements ensure that the chances of any kind of injury diminish considerably. At the same time within a short duration of practice benefits

begin to be visible. Even an extremely unfit individual who is not able to flex a particular muscle about a joint is able to see improvements with a couple of weeks itself. Whenever we utilize our muscles for some activity of daily life or for even exercise, there is a build up in the short term and some amount of residual accumulation in the long run of lactic acid, a waste product of anaerobic activity. This leads to stiffness, exhaustion, fatigue and pain. Through regular practice of yoga *asanas* dispersion of this lactic acid takes place.

Apart from the muscles in the body there are numerous other connective tissues such as ligaments and tendons. These tissues basically connect muscles and bones and also help control unwarranted movement of a joint above an acceptable range of motion. Athletes performing strenuous physical exercise and activities as well as general population are susceptible to injuries of these soft connective tissues. Yoga helps in increasing the mobility and flexibility of these tissues too and helps in preventing injuries. Improvement in range of motion about a joint and overall flexibility is by far the most commonly accepted reason as to why people start practicing yoga on a regular basis.

2. Strength – While practicing yoga, one is required to hold the various *asanas* or postures which required continuous recruitment of muscle fibers of various muscle groups. Numerous of these postures require load bearing of body weight which requires muscle contraction to take place. Simultaneously, to maintain balance in these postures neuromuscular coordination is required and that also recruits different muscle fibers. Overall strengthening of upper body, lower body and core takes place. This includes strengthening of not only major muscle groups such as shoulders, arms, hamstrings, quadriceps and abdominal group but also of smaller muscles of the back and neck, which prevent occurrences of common chronic ailments such as back pain and neck pain.

3. Posture – With increased flexibility and muscular strength, posture also improves. Almost all the standing as well as sitting exercises recruit and consequently strengthen the core muscles since they help in maintaining the poses for

longer periods of time. As a result of this posture improves drastically, and a person is able to sit, stand and walk in the correct posture. An increased level of awareness helps in correcting any slouch or slump. Most chronic muscular pains of the neck and back are a direct consequence of an inappropriate posture. By working on the source of the problem, yoga helps in eliminating these issues.

4. Weight loss – One of the most sought after benefits that pulls people towards yoga is weight loss. Yoga works on both sides of the problem, helps in reducing weight as well as works in reducing the tendency to gain weight. By working on physical aspects fat burning takes place during and after a yoga session. At the same time, by working on the mental aspects one is able to concentrate and adhere to weight loss plans by eating, thinking and resting healthy. Many forms of yoga involve fast, continuous and vigorous movement that helps to burn calories and thereby account for weight loss. We shall look at this aspect in detail in a subsequent section.

5. Breathing – A predominant component of yoga is *pranayama* or the set of breathing exercises that are performed. Deep and concentrated breathing helps improve lung capacity as well as respiratory rate. This is of immense importance during sports and endurance activities. A number of elite sports athletes nowadays are turning to yogic practices to improve their endurance and consequently athletic performance.

6. Cardiovascular endurance – 'Cardio' means heart and 'Vascular' means blood vessels. Together, 'Cardiovascular' system refers to the system in the body which provides oxygen to different parts of the body and helps utilize this oxygen to perform work. This includes involuntary activities such as beating of the heart controlled by the myocardial muscles as well as voluntary activities such as lifting a weight. All these activities require oxygen and the cardiovascular system is responsible for providing this efficiently. Yoga *asanas* help in lowering blood pressure levels and is immensely helpful in people having hypertension. It also helps in lowering the heart rate. Numerous studies have been conducted in this field, specially aiming to prove the positive effects of yoga on the cardiovascular system. Most of these studies provide a

direct positive correlation. Apart from this, there is significant evidence that yoga helps in lowering cholesterol and triglyceride levels in the blood. Certain forms of yoga such as power yoga involve fast, continuous movement through various *asanas* and are extremely useful in cardiovascular conditioning.

7. Improved immunity – Regular practice of yoga has also been seen to increase antioxidant levels resulting in improved immunity. Not only does this mean lesser susceptibility to illness but also a lower chance of getting these ailments and diseases in the first place, all because of a better immune system protecting the body.

8. Helps in injury rehabilitation – Forms of yoga such as *Iyengar yoga* involve slow and controlled movements. Postures are held in position for a brief while but for much longer a duration than normal. It is therefore easily performed by people beginning practice of yoga as well old people who are relatively unfit. Simultaneously, it is equally helpful for people who are recovering from injuries, specifically musculoskeletal injuries such as muscle pulls and repetitive stress injuries. Slow movements ensure that chances of injury are low and a person performs these *asanas* to the extent to which he or she is comfortable. The usage of props such as blocks, belts, blankets etc. make it easier for an individual to move closer to the perfect posture. Gradually the range of motion about joints increases as the injured soft tissues heal and become more and more flexible.

9. Improved bone mineral density – A number of yoga *asanas* are body weight bearing exercises. Our bones follow a rule, 'form follows function' which means that the more stress (under a particular range) that they undergo, the stronger they become. In such a manner yoga helps in increasing the bone mineral density. Post menopause women are susceptible to considerable loss of bone mineral and osteoporosis. Yoga helps prevent this loss of bone density.

10. Effects on medical conditions

    a. Migraine & headaches – Through an improved blood circulation and consequently better oxygen delivery to the brain, yoga helps in reducing and sometimes even eliminating the occurrences of headaches and migraines

b. Insomnia – People practicing yoga on a regular basis experience better, deeper and a more relaxed sleep. Problems such as insomnia are eliminates due to physiological benefits of yoga as well as psychological ones which lead to lower amounts of stress experienced

c. Treatment of cancer – Yoga is being increasingly used for treatment of cancer. It helps to decrease anxiety, pain and depression. Studies have found evidence that yoga leads to significantly lesser stress and mood disturbances as a result of which it is being used in cancer treatment

d. Yoga is also used in the treatment of schizophrenia where reduced stress and improved cognitive behavior lead to lower chances of relapse and better overall quality of life. Other chronic ailments for which yoga is used as a part of a comprehensive treatment plan include asthma, multiple sclerosis and arthritis

Psychological Benefits

1. Stress relief – Regular practice of yoga helps in getting stress levels down considerably. Even a regular 10 minute routine on a daily basis has shown to provide positive results. Yoga *asanas, pranayama* and meditation all help in relieving stress. In fact, yoga is incorporated as part of psychological therapy for treatment of stress related issues such as anxiety disorder and clinical depression.

2. Inner peace – Yoga helps in experiencing the inner peace within. A person does not have to depend on a vacation to go to a place that is away from the hustle & bustle of daily life. By practicing yoga one becomes aware of the immense peace that can be found within oneself. It is by far one of the best ways to calm a disturbed mind. It is in fact quite commonly used in helping people who have undergone some traumatic experience.

3. Greater awareness and observation – Due to the constant stresses of daily life, both at work and at home, one forgets to live in the present. Life is then dictated by what happens in the past and all our decisions are based on our self created image of the future. Yoga helps in understanding this very basic tendency of the mind. Through meditation it helps us in increasing our awareness and observation and helps us come back to the present. It helps us stay happy in the awareness of *what is* rather than worrying about *what can be.*
4. Increased energy levels – Even a short duration yoga session of only ten minutes helps one unwind. During the day when one feels energy sapped, yoga can help rejuvenate and reenergize within a few minutes. It thus gives us a feeling of renewed energy and acts like a energy booster in this regard
5. Better intuition – It has been experienced that yoga through its meditative component helps improve intuition. Belief in positive results helps us realize what is best and what needs to be done – our intuitive capabilities improve. It is not something that can be researched and scientifically proven in a laboratory. It needs to be believed in and experienced.

Concept of Weight Management

Before we discuss how yoga helps in weight management, a brief discussion on weight management is imperative. A program aimed at achieving and/or maintaining a particular body weight is known as a weight management program. In general, this can be divided into two categories, weight gain and weight loss program.

Body Composition

The human body is composed of bones, lean muscle, fat, organs and water along with other parts such as skin, hair etc. Through a weight management program we aim to alter the body weight by altering either the lean muscle mass or the fat mass in the body. As is apparent the other constituent elements are not tampered with within the context of a weight management program. There are many methods to determine the amounts or percentages of different constituent elements in the body. Traditionally skin–fold measurements using calipers have been used for determining fat percentage. However, this method is slightly inaccurate and also does not provide a complete picture. Over the years numerous technologies have come into the forefront, which provide accurate and complete results in a matter of a few seconds. The commonly used ones include Ultrasound and Bio–electric Impedance Analysis.

Weight Loss Versus Weight Gain

When the goal is to lose weight, the aim is to cut down on the fat mass. Fat is present in the body under the skin, also known as subcutaneous fat; and also around the organs predominantly in the abdominal region, this is known as visceral fat. When we lose fat, we lose it from all over the body and not from one targeted specific area. This is so because fat is an energy substrate that is used for metabolic purposes equal proportion from all areas of the body. The goal is to ensure that to meet the energy requirements of the body, whether it is for activities of daily life or for exercise, the energy is provided by burning the fat that is stored in the body. The goal is thus to lose weight by losing fat while maintaining or increasing lean muscle tissue.

When the goal is weight gain, the aim is to increase the lean muscle mass in the body and to cut down on the fat percentage. Gaining muscle mass is done through anabolic processes o growth processes. Lean muscle is gained through a combination of right exercise specifically resistance training along with the right kind of diet, which provides the body with the necessary fuel to grow. Contrary to weight loss, lean muscle tissue can be gained in specific areas of the body. By working out or exercising the muscles of the lower body, lean muscle tissue will be added to the muscle groups of the legs such as quadriceps, hamstrings and calves. By working out on the muscles of the upper body, lean muscle tissue will be added to the chest, shoulders, biceps, triceps and forearms. Within each of these muscle groups there are individual muscles that can be worked out by performing a whole variety of exercises. Except when a person is severely underweight with little fat in the body, generally fat is limited to a certain percentage. In a normal healthy male fat percentage should be around 10 – 15% while that in women it should be around 20 -25%. This is so because even fat has many important functions in the body such as thermo regulation, cushioning and protection of organs, and as an efficient energy store.

Healthy Weight Management

Healthy weight management is a multifaceted concept that is done in a gradual manner. The four pillars of wellness are physical exercise, diet & nutrition, rest & mental relaxation and attitude. Weight loss done in a way that ignores any particular aspect of wellness will invariably lead to sub-optimal results. For example, a weight management program that concentrates only on diet will help the individual to lose weight; but the weight loss thus achieved will include loss of lean muscle tissue as well which is undesirable.

Secondly, the rate at which weight loss or gain happens is also very important. In an effort to lose weight fast individuals get carried away at times and lose weight too fast. This is also not desired since the different systems of the body such as cardiovascular system, hormonal system etc. are used to functioning in a particular manner for the specific body type. Sudden changes are not well adapted by these systems as a result of which there are chances that some complications may arise. A good benchmark is loss or gain of 1 to 2 pounds of body weight per week. This gives time to the body to make necessary adjustments. Weight management done in this particular manner is considered healthy.

Yoga through different *asanas* that resemble body weighted exercises provides resistance training to different muscle groups. By performing particular *asanas* that target specific muscle groups we can increase the lean muscle tissue mass for muscles of that group. In such a way yoga can help in healthy weight gain that is through an increase in lean mass. In the following section though, the problem of weight loss has been catered to since the positive psychological effects that yoga has is applicable to weight gain programs in almost exactly the same way.

Benefits of Yoga In Relation to Weight Loss

One of the most widely accepted benefits of yoga is that it helps in healthy weight management. Not only does it work on the physical aspects of weight loss but also helps in tuning the mental faculties in a positive manner such that weight loss is facilitated. Since yoga promotes healthy weight loss, it is sustainable unlike unhealthy methods such as crash dieting.

Weight Loss – Background

A person can be overweight due to numerous reasons such as physiological, psychological, social and cultural factors. Whereas, certain lifestyle patterns are easier to alter leading to weight loss, there are other physiological parameters such as hormonal issues and psychological parameters such as emotional issues like depression and anxiety disorders; these may pose significantly greater problems in achieving weight loss. These emotional complications lead to people having literally no control over their dietary habits, emotional eating may follow which leads to weight gain. Even those who go on strict dietary regimens like crash diets are prone to gaining the lost weight back again. Even if they see results for a while, it is highly probable that they lose focus at some time and the binge eating that follows causes them to gain back all the lost weight. Obesity can be chronic in which a person keeps gaining weight steadily and continuously; it can also be fluctuating in nature, wherein a person gains and looses weight in a fluctuating manner.

How Yoga Works

As seen above, there are many reasons for a person gaining weight. Yoga is extremely efficient in weight loss since it provides a multi–faceted approach; it does not work on the symptoms alone, but targets the root cause or core of the problem. It takes into account physical, emotional and mental components in dealing with the problem. Losing weight through yoga involves improving cardiovascular endurance, detoxification, increasing the metabolic rate, improving focus and awareness of goals and attaining appropriate hormonal balance. Practice of certain forms of yoga which are extremely fast paced and vigorous in nature resembles a cardiovascular endurance workout. There is hardly any gap between two *asanas* or postures, as a result of which the heart rate increases and is maintained at these high levels during the entire session. In such a manner, forms of yoga such as *Power yoga* and *Bikram yoga* are more efficient in comparison to forms such as *Iyengar yoga*. Practice of *kriyas* such as *surya namaskar* and *kapal bhati* done at a fast pace provide a decent cardiovascular workout.

Through different *asanas* specific training of different parts of the body can be performed. It is believed that flexion of the trunk brings about a certain amount of calmness while extension of the trunk leads to boosting of energy in the body. Practice of *pranayama* leads to a reduction in anxiety, helps in detoxifying the body and also increases metabolism. It also helps in an increased capacity of the body to transport essential nutrients and oxygen to different parts of the body where they can be utilized effectively. Yoga also effects the secretion of hormones from the thyroid and pituitary glands, which brings about a balance in the hormonal system and consequently positively affects the metabolic rate. *Pranayama* and meditation provide a calming influence over the mind. There is an increase in awareness of the present and this helps in improving focus. In such a way yoga helps in increasing adherence to the weight loss program. It also enforces the link between mind & body. One becomes more aware of the present, of what is being eaten and when the body feels full. This understanding is important in creating an environment where healthy eating is promoted and is sustainable. It is not based on the fabric of denial, which is bound to fail either today or tomorrow.

Weight loss is a complex problem and therefore the solution cannot be one–dimensional. Just working on calorie intake or burning calories through intense long duration workouts will not provide a sustainable solution. Yoga on the contrary works in a holistic manner. The attempt is towards creating a harmony between mind, body & soul. The entire exercise is looked at positively rather than as a punishment through which the body needs to be put for attaining weight loss. It is the entire process of the present that becomes enjoyable and this positivity ensures weight loss results.

Precautions To Be Considered While Performing Yoga

Yoga is an extremely safe practice. However, risks present themselves specifically when without adequate knowledge people start performing complex *asanas*. The following precautions need to be taken before beginning the practice of Yoga:

1. It is recommended to consult a doctor or physician before starting any kind of yogic practice in case of severe conditions of osteoporosis, spine related problems, hypertension and also in case of pregnancy.

2. It is highly recommended that yoga be learnt under the supervision of a learned instructor. It may seem easy to follow books and online tutorials, but if improperly performed may be risky.
3. Understand your body and know the limits to which it can be stretched. The body should not be pushed to an extent where chances of injury become high. For example there may be a slight discomfort such as a mild stretch that may be experienced while performing a particular *asana*; this is fine. However, there should be no pain whatsoever. In case this happens then it is highly recommended to stop immediately before an injury occurs.
4. It is important to go slow and at a steady pace that is comfortable for the body. In group classes there is a tendency to push beyond acceptable limits, so that synchronization with the group is maintained. It is recommended that yoga should be practiced at a pace where one is comfortable. Since it is not a race, there is no reason why more time cannot be devoted to learning a particular aspect that may perhaps be difficult to grasp.

Yoga is not a pill that will provide instant results. It is a way of life; a holistic practice that improves all aspects of life and creates harmony between the body, mind and soul.

Lifestyle Diary

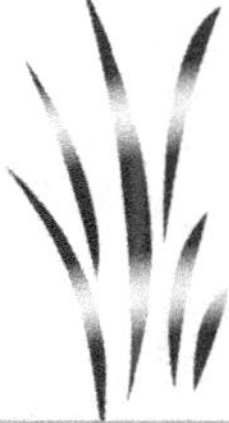

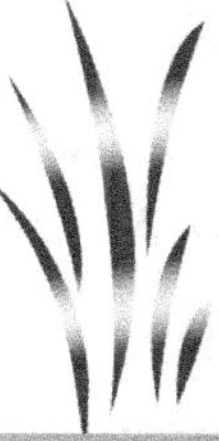

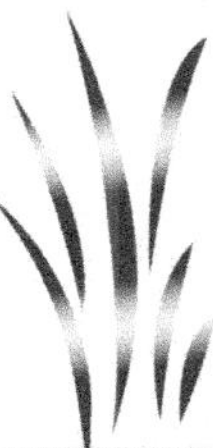

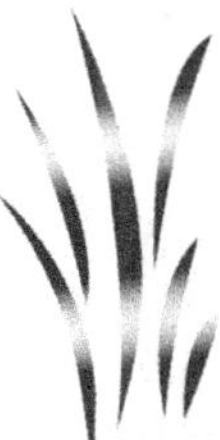

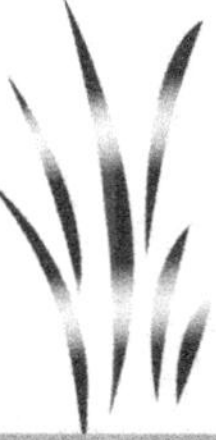

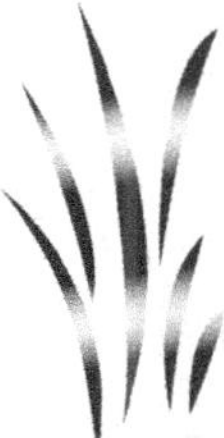

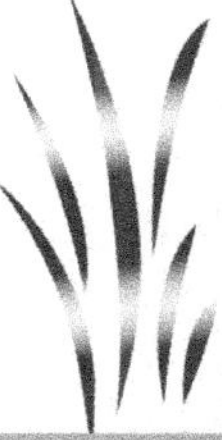

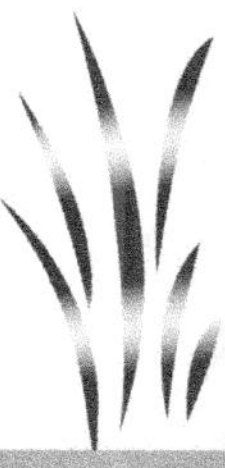

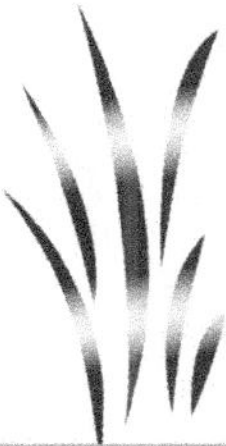

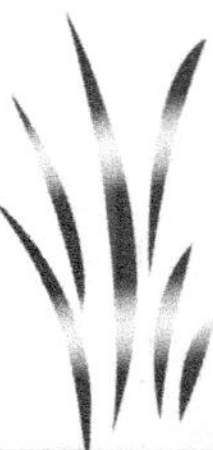

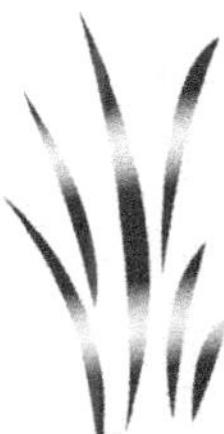

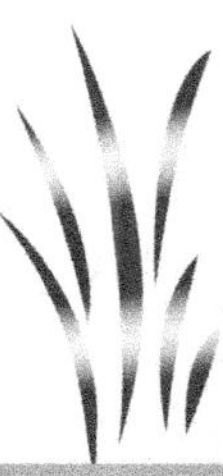

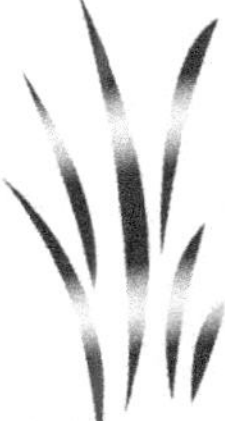

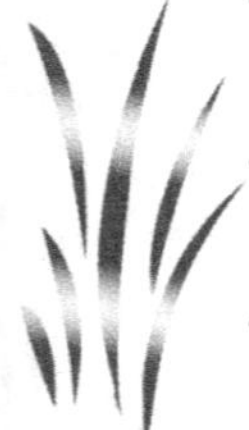

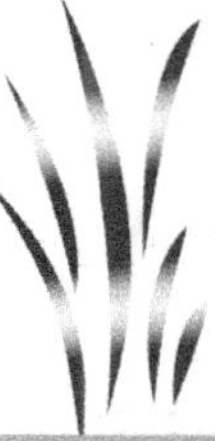

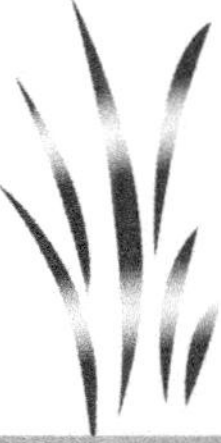

Also Available From Innovative Publishers

Introduction to the Paleo diet.

Introduction to the Paleo diet (includes 200 recipes).

Love is…

Extreme Betrayal

Beware the Bumble Bee

Doing business with the government.

Visit http://innovative-publishers.com for ordering information

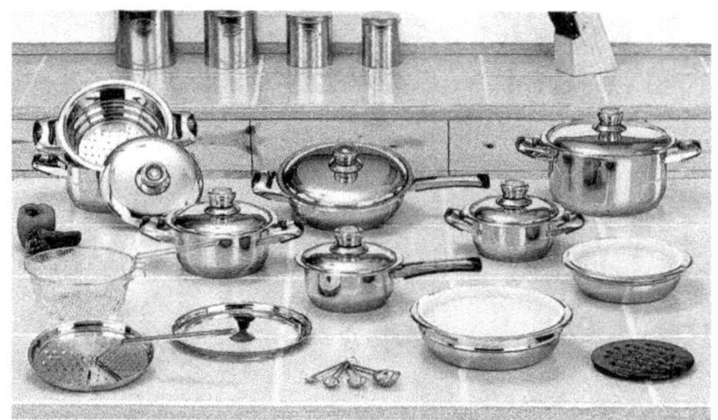

28pc 12-Element High-Quality, Heavy-Gauge Stainless Steel Cookware Set

This set does it all! Now you can have the perfect pan for any cooking job and the right accessories to help you prepare meals like a professional chef. The unique temperature knob on each cover tells you when you have reached the optimum temperature for healthy and nutrient-saving waterless cooking. More than high-quality cookware, each accessory offers greater efficiency and usefulness. The high-quality stainless steel bowls can also be used as double boilers or even as dome covers for stove-top roasting. The handy step-steamer lets you steam just the right quantity of vegetables because it fits the saucepan and 4 sizes of casseroles. Each pan is made from beautifully polished, high-quality stainless steel together with high-quality stainless steel capped, riveted handles for durability and performance that will last a lifetime. Set includes: 1.6qt saucepan with cover, 1.6qt casserole with cover, 2.2qt casserole with cover, 3.1qt casserole with cover, step-steamer with side handles, 6qt casserole with cover, 10-7/8" frypan with cover, large mixing bowl with airtight plastic cover, medium mixing bowl with airtight plastic cover, grater with removable handle, grater ring adapter, deep fry basket with removable handle, suction cup knob for mixing bowls when used as a dome cover, heat-resistant pan rest, and 4pc measuring spoons. Limited lifetime warranty. Gift boxed.

Suggested Retail Price : $1100.00
Your price: 70% OFF + shipping

Item Number : GGKT28

Set Contents

- 1.6Qt Saucepan With Cover
- 1.6Qt Casserole With Cover
- 2.2Qt Casserole With Cover
- 3.1Qt Casserole With Cover
- Step-Steamer With Side Handles
- 6Qt Casserole With Cover
- 10-7/8" Edge To Edge Frypan With Cover
- Large Mixing Bowl With Airtight Plastic Cover
- Medium Mixing Bowl With Airtight Plastic Cover
- Grater With Removable Handle
- Grater Ring Adapter
- Deep Fry Basket With Removable Handle
- Suction Cup Knob For Mixing Bowls When Used As A Dome Cover
- Heat-Resistant Pan Rest
- 4Pc Measuring Spoons

Features

- 12-Element Construction
- Encapsulated Bottom For Even Heat Distribution
- Mirror Finish Interior & Exterior
- Thermo Top Knobs
- Riveted, Heat-Resistant Phenolic/Metal Handles
- Limited Lifetime Warranty

» Estimated Case Dimensions : 22.59" Length, 20.23" Width, 8.25" Height

» Estimated Case Weight : 28.65 Lbs.

To order, go to http://groupglobal.net/ and click on retail shopping.

Coupon Code: GGKT28-70

About the Author

C. T. Pam is not a physician, rather she is a regular person who has explored many avenues of eating healthy and finding a healthy lifestyle balance. After a car accident in 2010 left her unable to continue running, she found a work-life balance that has helped her maintain a healthy lifestyle. C. T. Pam has a B.A. in Political Science and Studio Art, an MBA with a entrepreneurship concentration and is currently pursuing a doctoral degree with a research focus in Entrepreneurship.

www.ingramcontent.com/pod-product-compliance
Lightning Source LLC
La Vergne TN
LVHW010059110826
845155LV00028B/403

* 9 7 8 1 8 8 4 7 1 1 3 4 3 *